Kaizen-durance
Book One

SHANE EVERSFIELD

CONTENTS

ACKNOWLEDGMENTS

Text and concept: Shane Eversfield

Cover Design and Graphic Artwork: Mat Hudson

© Kaizen-durance

First edition published 2017.

CHAPTER ONE:
THE ENDURANCE ATHLETE'S DILEMMA

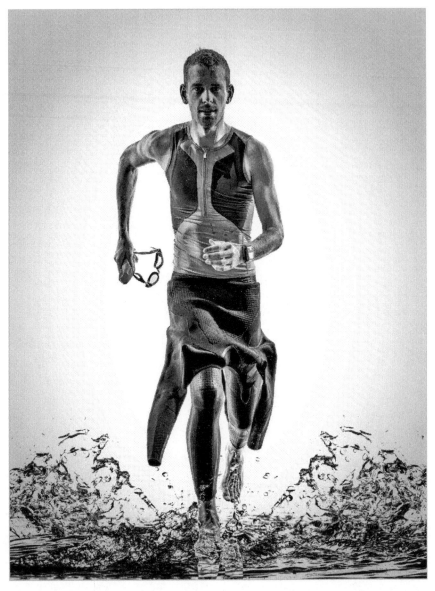

The Aerobic Wall

Are you an *aging* athlete?

If you *are* an athlete, but you are *not* aging, put this book down right now and contact me! I want to know your secret.

If you *are* an aging athlete, 28 years of age or older, here's something you may want to consider: Your aerobic potential is declining. That is, your cardiovascular system is past its prime.

Imagine your aerobic capacity as a wall. Once you reach 28 years of age, that wall starts advancing towards you. Sure, we all hope that the advance is slow. And conventional endurance training focuses almost entirely on slowing the inevitable advance of that Aerobic Wall.

We may slow that advance with relentless and diligent training - often at the risk of injury or illness. But… we cannot stop it from encroaching on our performance.

What do we get for all of that perseverance? Sometimes it just feels like we're just banging our heads against the Aerobic Wall. After a few years, or perhaps a few decades, many of us simply resign. Often with battle scars from slamming ourselves against that advancing wall: chronic joint injuries, chronic endocrine/adrenal fatigue, heart disease, failed marriages, despair, boredom, burnout…

Even if we meticulously follow the very latest groundbreaking scientifically-based training protocols, even if we consume the best supplements and fuels, all of us continue to age… and slow down.

Is it possible for us as aging endurance athletes to experience growth, progress and satisfaction in our pursuits *even as that Aerobic Wall encroaches upon us?*

As I approach 60 years of age, I am continuing to complete events that are longer and more challenging than when I was younger. And while I am slowing down, I am also experiencing more grace and finesse in the same events I have competed in for decades. Most remarkable to me, I am also recovering *faster.*

The growth and discovery I am enjoying now are *not* the result of magic or good luck. Instead, I am successfully navigating the path of Kaizen-durance. You too can continue to enjoy growth, progress and satisfaction - not just in athletics, but in every area of your life - without continuing to bang your head against that Aerobic Wall.

So, where do we start? Let's begin with…

Effortless Power

At the risk of dating myself here (after all, I am an aging athlete): Do you recall the TV show "Kung Fu"? Or, perhaps you remember the movie "Karate Kid"? Each of these depicts a wise old oriental sage who appears feeble and vulnerable. In Kung Fu, the sage is even *blind.* In Karate Kid, he seems a bit crazy.

And yet, when a brash young warrior attacks the sage, he calmly and effortlessly neutralizes his would-be assailant - even the most robust and muscular. He does this without exertion or force of his own. This frail master seems to possess some kind of mysterious "effortless power". And, this effortless power appears to grow stronger with age.

This effortless power the wise old master demonstrates, it is a myth, or is it real?

Kaizen

Kaizen is a Japanese word derived from the Chinese "Gai Shan". Kaizen translates as "lifelong improvement".

It's no coincidence that the expression "Kaizen" and the image of the wise old sage both arise from the Orient. The questions for us are:

- Is Kaizen - this "lifelong improvement" - possible for us as aging endurance athletes?

- Can our advancing age account for something besides aerobic decline?

- Is there some kind of "endurance wisdom" we can accrue, like the mysterious effortless power of those legendary oriental masters of the martial arts?

- Is there a kaizen path we can follow that will lead us towards "endurance wisdom"?

- A wisdom that enables us to discover, articulate and enjoy our own form of effortless power in endurance sports?

Kaizen-durance

The answer is YES. The effortless power we dream of lies hidden within the pursuit of Kaizen-durance.

There are some legends in the arena of endurance sports that demonstrate Kaizen-durance and defy our conventions about aging. Guy Rossi is one of those. He is 78 years old, and still doing double irons. (That's double the distance of an iron triathlon.) He has finished: 69 doubles, 27 triples, 4 quintuples, and 10 deca-irons. Along with his single irons, he has done a total of 343 irons since he began in 1985.

In this book, we explore the foundational elements of Kaizen-durance and how we can forge skills for lifelong improvement from these foundations. As we train each day, we can develop these kaizen skills even as we continue to pursue our highest endurance goals.

Even more promising and rewarding: Well beyond our lives as an endurance athletes, we can use these same skills to enhance and enrich our relationships with family and friends, our occupations, and any visions we have for our lives.

Our daily endurance training offers us a golden opportunity to develop kaizen skills for lifelong growth and improvement. Let's do more with our passion for endurance sports than bang our heads against the "Aerobic Wall".

No longer are we required to be the "aging athlete". From now on, we can choose to be the "master athlete".

CHAPTER TWO:

FITNESS CYCLE: THE WHEEL OF LIFE

The Fitness Cycle

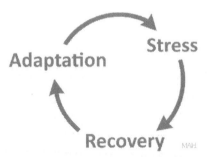

Fitness Cycle

Stress-Recovery-Adaptation:

The Fitness Cycle has three phases: Stress, Recovery and Adaptation.

If we turn the wheel of the Fitness Cycle over and over in a well-chosen direction, we can roll forward in our preparation for the next goal race. We train, we recover, we get stronger. That's one revolution of the wheel. The more we turn the wheel, the further and faster we can progress.

However…

If we try to turn the wheel too fast, and it gets away from us, we lose control and crash. Then, we can't move forward again until we repair the wheel - get it true and balanced - so we can roll it forward again. When we train too hard, too long and/or too frequently, we turn the wheel too fast. The crash occurs when we get injured, sick or burned out.

If we turn the wheel too slow, it simply stops and falls over. No forward movement here either, until we get the wheel upright, aimed in the intended direction, and rolling fast enough to keep gyroscopic balance. When we train too easy, too briefly and/or inconsistently we turn the wheel too slow. The wheel falls over when we get sedentary, distracted or lose motivation.

Gimme the Stress!

As endurance athletes, we like the feeling of accomplishment that comes with training. *"I ran 10K this morning over hilly terrain. Then I swam 18 X 100 meters after work."* Many of us invest lots of time and energy carefully designing and executing very specific workouts. Or we hire a coach to do it for us. But remember, these workouts are just *one phase* of the Fitness Cycle: the Stress Phase. During this phase we are actually orchestrating *damage* to our bodies. If we orchestrate this phase correctly, the damage is incremental, and not catastrophic.

As endurance athletes, many of us do not feel the same sense of accomplishment that comes with Recovery or Adaptation. The recovery process just doesn't fit our popular image of the endurance athlete: The scantily dressed, focus-driven, forward-surging gladiator. Consequently, we are less invested and deliberate about these two Phases of the Fitness Cycle. However, if we don't balance the Stress with adequate and effective Recovery and Adaptation, we lose control of the wheel of our Fitness Cycle.

To summarize, we need Stress to stimulate growth: No stress equals couch potato. However, without Recovery and Adaptation, we won't realize that growth: No recovery equals burned out.

Three Physiological Systems

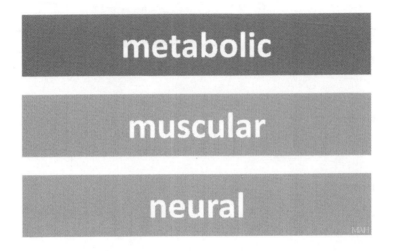

Training: Behind the Scenes

Let's look a little deeper now at exactly what we are "damaging" when we train.

As athletes, we train three physiological systems: muscular, metabolic, neurological. In conventional "Energy System Training" (EST), we design our workouts primarily to stress and improve the metabolic system. When we stress the metabolic system, it damages the metabolic components of our cells.

Your metabolic system determines your aerobic fitness. Remember that Aerobic Wall from the Introduction? Here it is: EST tasks us to push relentlessly against that encroaching Aerobic Wall. *"Don't stop pushing! Maybe you can slow down the advance!"*

If we damage this system too severely when we train, we increase our risk of injury, sickness, endocrine/adrenal fatigue, cardiac arrest, etc. This also affects our temperament and performance in every area of life. While we are striving for our maximum aerobic potential, we may compromise our health and well-being.

A peaked, super-fit athlete is not necessarily a healthy human being.

Here's a powerful question that may change the focus of our training: What physiological system can respond and improve the most to training over the long-term? It's not our metabolic system. And it's not our muscular system.

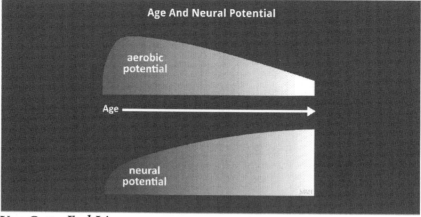

You Gotta *Feel It!*

Our *neural* system can respond and improve the most to endurance training. While the Aerobic Wall advances towards us as we age, there is no "Neural Wall". (At least not for those of us who are free from any neurological diseases such as A.L.S. or M.S.) While our metabolic potential is diminishing with age, our neural potential remains strong, at least into our seventies, or even our *eighties or beyond.*

(Note: Throughout the Kaizen-durance series of books, I will use the term *"neural"* rather than *"nervous"*. I have chosen this to avoid the association between the nervous system and the condition of nervousness.)

As master athletes, our path to Kaizen is through *neural fitness.* I am not declaring that we should ignore the pursuit of metabolic health and aerobic fitness. But, if we ignore neural fitness, then we are aiming the wheel of our Fitness Cycle directly towards that Aerobic Wall. Every time we hit that wall, we risk injury, sickness and burnout. If instead we aim the wheel towards neural fitness, there is no wall, no limit, no impact. We can roll forward for a very long time.

Metabolic potential is a diminishing resource for the aging athlete. Neural potential is an abundant resource for the master athlete.

Looking for proof? Consider the Hawaii Ironman World Championship, pinnacle in the sport of triathlon. For over three decades, athletes - both male and female - have strived to become one of the legends of the Kona lava fields. They train meticulously for years, sacrificing and investing heavily to vie for the coveted *"Haku Lei"* crown at the finish line.

The winners each year are *consistently in their early-to-mid-thirties.* Paula Newby-

Fraser won her eighth World Championship at age *forty*. (That's two more times than the top males; Mark Allen and Dave Scott each won six times.) But how can this be? These champions are years - perhaps a decade or more - beyond aerobic prime.

While virtually all of these athletes focus on aerobic fitness, they are also improving their *neural* fitness. For these World Champions, the decline in aerobic fitness is more than compensated by their increase in *neural fitness*. I call this long-term build of neural fitness *"kinetic intelligence"*. (We will explore kinetic intelligence in Chapter 4.)

In simplest terms, when we train neural fitness, we *move smarter*. We are able to swim, bike and run farther and/or faster with less energy, less injury and faster recovery. We rely far less on the high-tech instruments that measure heart rate, power output and pace because we are more in tune with the most intelligent instrument of all - *our own bodies*.

What happens when we begin to patiently focus on training neural fitness and developing kinetic intelligence? We can defy our own perceived limits:

Twelve years ago (age forty-seven), I had been through chronic adrenal fatigue three times. I decided to stop banging my head so hard against that Aerobic Wall. When I began to focus on neural training and kinetic intelligence, I had no idea what I would accomplish in my fifties:

- Eighth in age group at ITU Long Course Triathlon World Championship (2008)

- Multiple double and triple irons and Ultramans

- Consecutive weekends of ultra running from marathons to hundred-milers (up to 4 weeks in a row).

- A one hundred mile mountain bike race. (With minimal mountain bike technique.)

- Rapid recovery, and almost zero injuries

All of this on an average of 14 hours per week of training. I'm looking forward to what unfolds *in my sixties!*

Self-Evaluation

Here are a few questions you can ask yourself:

- Are you balancing the Stress of your training sessions with adequate Recovery and Adaptation?

- Do you design and execute your Recovery with the same diligence as the Stress?

- Do you keep a training journal?

Important to remember: Stress is stress. If you are experiencing stress in other areas of your life, *you may need to ease up on the stress of athletic training.* Our body's endocrine system doesn't care if if the source of stress is from endurance training, or some other area of life. Stress is stress.

Log your Training *and your Recovery Indicators*:

Check your resting heart rate each morning when you wake up, before you get out of bed. An elevated resting heart rate can indicate that you are not yet recovered. Its normal to experience this for a day or two after a particularly challenging session. However, if it's elevated for several days in a row, you are at risk.

Track your moods each day. Watch for:

- Impatience with other people or yourself

- A lack of enthusiasm for training

- Appetite: Lack of appetite can indicate lack of recovery

Monitor sleep quality and amount. Watch for:

- You go to bed exhausted and then wake up an hour or two later unable to sleep

- You are restless and jumpy throughout the night

- You find it very difficult to wake up and get out of bed

Monitor caffeine intake: Do you rely heavily and consistently on caffeine to stay functional and motivated?

Watch for chronic inflammation and weight fluctuations

Zenman's Recovery

Here are four effective practices you can implement to bring mastery to your recovery process:

1) Recline and Reset:

Lie down for 10-20 minutes. Breathe slow and deep as you relax your body. We will explore the "Body Scan" - a more advanced process for this - in Chapter 6. To maximize the benefits of Recline and Reset:

- If possible do this in a dark, quiet space. You can simply cover your eyes, and use ear plugs if necessary.

- Coordinate your Recline and Reset soon after your training to optimize the recovery effect. Or, you can set aside 10 minutes of your lunch break on work days. If you are consistent about the timing of your Recline and Reset, your mind and body will learn to "navigate" this process well to optimize the benefits.

Mastering Recline and Reset is just as valuable as mastering your swimming, biking, running, etc.

2) Nutrition for Recovery:

When you finish your training, refuel within 20 minutes. Ingest about 200 calories and some form of protein. Find a refuel protocol that serves your body well. Advice from the experts varies widely on this. Educate yourself, but ultimately: *Trust your own body.* That is, *listen* to your body. As you develop this valuable listening skill, you can hone in on exactly what is right for you.

Your overall diet also has a profound impact on how well you recover from *all* forms of stress. Some foods will add stress to your life. Others will support recovery. Again, educate yourself, but ultimately: *Trust what your body says.*

3) Active Recovery:

Research shows that novice endurance athletes benefit best from "total rest days" - that is passive days with no endurance training at all. It also shows that seasoned athletes usually benefit best from "*active* recovery" - that is, days with easy, gentle exercise. The master athlete has the *patience* to conduct active recovery training sessions that accelerate recovery without adding more stress.

To master the art of Active Recovery, you must be willing to "let go of the numbers": Gently engage in some form of easy exercise without any fixation on a pace or distance. Typically, 20-40 minutes is adequate. If you are a single-sport athlete, your ideal form of active recovery may be some activity other than your chosen sport.

We will explore further the Golden Opportunity of active recovery in Chapter 4.

4) Daily Gratitudes:

Take time each day - even just a few moments - to reflect on what you are grateful for in your life. Ideally, these gratitudes should include elements of all areas of your life - not just your athletic life. Your gratitudes can include the *challenges* that you are experiencing in any area of your life. When we embrace the challenges of our lives as opportunities for growth, we are more apt to roll the wheel of the Fitness Cycle forward. Remember, this Fitness Cycle is the Wheel of Life, not just athletics.

Chapter Summary

- The Fitness Cycle has three phases: Stress, Recovery and Adaptation.

- To train effectively we need to balance these three phases and move through the cycle at an appropriate speed.

- As endurance athletes, it's easy for us to focus on the Stress phase, because that phase occurs during our actual training. We are often less diligent about orchestrating our Recovery Adaptation.

- We need stress to stimulate growth. We need recovery and adaptation to actually realize it.

- We train three physiological systems: muscular, metabolic, neurological. Conventional training and coaching focuses on training the metabolic through Energy System Training.

- Metabolic potential is a diminishing resource for the aging athlete.

Neural potential is an abundant resource for the master athlete.

- Four effective practices to optimize recovery: Recline and Reset, Nutrition for Recovery, Active Recovery, Daily Gratitudes.

What's Next?

In the next chapter, we will look deeper into Kaizen: what it is and how to activate it our lives.

CHAPTER THREE:

THE PURSUIT OF MASTERY

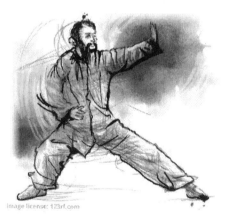

Image license: 123rf.com

All Grown Up Now?

For some of us, being an adult is synonymous with being a *grown-up*. A grown-up has reached the ceiling: Nothing more to learn, nothing else to explore: *"Been there, done that, period."*

The possibility of kaizen - lifelong improvement - defies our convention of "grown up". As adults, we are compelled to fulfill our familial, occupational and civic responsibilities. However, that does not mean that we have to terminate our growth and learning. In each moment of our daily lives, we have the opportunity to pursue mastery. Kaizen does not mean that we have to compromise the responsibilities of adulthood. Instead, these responsibilities are rich opportunities for the pursuit of mastery.

So, What is Mastery?

Let's return to the image of the wise old martial arts master. This master responds to his opponent with ease. He moves with grace and harmony, welcoming each challenge from his opponent.

Without the insightful skills of mastery, we are prone to struggle and resist the challenges in our lives. We experience these challenges as confrontations that threaten our well-being, our comfort. As we acquire the insights and skills of the master, we welcome and embrace these challenges as opportunities - even if we don't *like* them.

These challenges that arise in our lives - in every area of our lives - they are forms of stress. They are part of that Fitness Cycle, that Wheel of Life. Without the skills of mastery, we push back at these challenges - just like we have been taught to bang our heads against the Aerobic Wall. Rather than responding, we react. Our resistance and reaction *actually magnify the stress*, often beyond our ability to readily recover and adapt. Now the Wheel of Life is rolling backwards, and our health is compromised by chronic stress, and the absence of recovery and adaptation.

Mastery empowers us to *respond*, rather than react. The difference between the two is subtle, yet very profound. Without mastery the Wheel of Life either falls over or moves backwards. With mastery, we roll the Wheel of Life forward, *and* we choose the direction it moves.

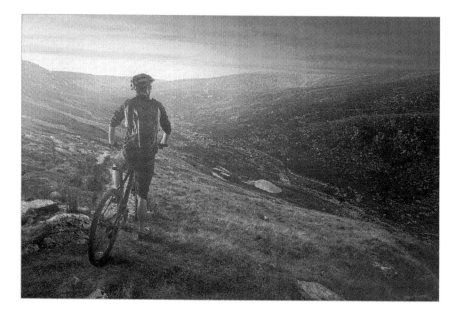

Here's the "Catch"

In the pursuit of mastery, *there is no glorious finish line*. After all, we're talking about life-long improvement. Our pursuit continues until we die.

"Really, no finish line? So what's the point?"

Recall one of your most significant endurance races: When you register for this event, you probably begin to imagine the finish line - how you will feel crossing that line, receiving your medal, enjoying the relief and finally being able to rest. Next, you invest months of your time and energy preparing for this event so that you can wear that medal. Your focus is the finish.

Now, suppose you could simply *buy* the medal and the finisher's shirt - without the investment of time and energy to train. Not good enough? How about if you could start just 100 yards away and dash down the finisher's chute with the same fanfare, receiving the same genuine recognition and respect from everyone? Would it feel the same for you, even if everything on the "outside" was identical in your finish line scenario? Do you feel some aversion now for this scenario?

If so, your motivation to register for that challenging event, and to diligently prepare for months to complete it is not just for the accolades and glory of the finish line. There's more to it than a few moments of acclaim, and the sparkle of that weighty finisher's medal. Perhaps it really is about the journey - about the challenges, experiences and insights you move through along the way to that finish line. Perhaps it's about the pursuit of mastery.

Sure, as master athletes, we do pause occasionally to reflect on how that brief moment of finish line glory felt, to enjoy the collection of medals, awards and shirts we have earned. However, it's the experiences of our endurance lifestyle that are a *living part of our being* - these are the most precious rewards.

While the pursuit of mastery may not have an absolute finish line, we do traverse incredible landscapes, through all kinds of weather (emotional, mental and physical) as we forge ahead in that endless pursuit. The experiences - both high and low - are deep and rich.

An endurance event can feel like an analogy for life. In life, do we charge for the "finish line" as quickly as possible, with as much effort, discomfort and struggle as we can muster? Perhaps a more satisfying and enriching life arises when we fully experience and engage in each moment of the journey, each relationship, each task that arises - without the hurry to get it all over with.

The Paradox of Control

That wise old martial arts master does not attempt to *control* his opponent. Instead, he patiently engages and *plays* with his opponent's force. In this way, he can channel and redirect his opponent's force while conserving his own need to generate force. In this way, he fights using *effortless power*. He draws upon the forces that are already "at play".

Our wise sensei cannot control his opponent any more than we can control the circumstances or relationships of our lives. He surrenders his attachment to dominate his opponent. Instead, he opens up to the opportunities that arise in each moment.

This can be confusing: Surrendering control, but still pursuing mastery? How can we get anything done in life if we are completely passive and submissive?

The distinction is subtle. The sensei is still pursuing a result, but he has given up his *attachment* for that result. He is patient, and focuses on what is unfolding here and now, without struggling to control the outcome. As master athletes, we too can give up our attachment to the finish line result.

This frees up our energy to train effectively today using the circumstances that are unfolding here and now.

The Paradox of Control may be confusing. That's the nature of a *paradox*. No worries, we will explore this paradox throughout the Kaizen-durance book series.

What Makes a Master?

What does the master do to pursue mastery and enjoy this effortless power? What does s/he possess that others don't?

The master is committed to finding an opportunity for growth and improvement in every moment, every circumstance, every relationship, every task. Ideally, she seeks that opportunity regardless of her likes or dislikes, opinions or judgments, desires, fears, etc. about the circumstance, relationship or task. She experiences growth and improvement in each moment through one very simple, yet highly challenging commitment: The master relentlessly strives for *perceptive acuity*. That is, we gain proficiency (mastery) as we more accurately perceive what is occurring in the present moment.

As a *teacher*, the master does not actually teach. She simply encourages her student to *be more perceptive*.

We have all heard the expression *"Pay attention!"* Paying infers that we are losing something or clearing a debt. Instead, perceptive acuity requires that we *invest* our awareness and attention. Investment infers that we are choosing to contribute our assets (in this case our awareness and attention) towards something. We invest our awareness and attention for perceptive clarity, accuracy. Now we can fully engage in life.

Recalling the TV show "Kung Fu", the feeble looking old master is *blind*. Yet, he can still accurately perceive and deftly respond to his opponents. OK, so that's a TV show… How about a real-life example?

No Limits

Helen Keller was both blind and deaf from birth. That's like being in solitary confinement beginning at birth. Despite such profound limitations, with the patient support and assistance of Annie Sullivan, Helen lived a rich and fulfilling life. She made a difference the world over, despite such a minuscule portal with the outside world.

Helen Keller's greatest contribution to humanity? She demonstrated for us that there are simply *no limits* to either our perceptive capacity, or our expressive capacity. Without sight or sound, she still lived a life rich with experience. With Annie's love and relentless commitment, Helen transformed the rage and groundless isolation of her lonely childhood into creative vision and expression that continues to inspire us today.

Helen Keller's message to all of us is this: There are *no limits to our experience-ability.* That is:

- No limits to our awareness and attention.

- No limits to how much and how deeply we can invest.

Our infinite experience-ability empowers each of us to kaizen. There are no limits and so there is no absolute finish line.

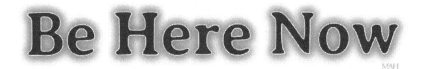

Be Here Now

However... Our infinite ability to perceive and express *is limited* in one way: It exists *only in this present moment.* It does not exist in the past or in the future. If we constantly dwell in the past or live only for the future, we have no investment opportunity. The pursuit of mastery can only occur *here and now.*

It requires rigorous training for us to Be Here Now - to consistently and patiently return our attention to this present moment every time it wanders off. Indeed, this training to Be Here Now in the present moment of our lives is more rigorous and challenging than training for an iron triathlon.

However, as endurance athletes, we have the opportunity to train and develop the essential skills that do enable us to Be Here Now, so that we can fully invest our attention and awareness and enjoy lifelong improvement. These essential skills are called *"mindfulness skills"*. We can develop these mindfulness skills *at the same time* we are training as endurance athletes.

As master athletes, these mindfulness skills will improve our athletic performance. It's all about fully investing our attention in what we are doing, feeling, thinking and saying... here and now. Train better. Race better. Live better.

What Are Your Opportunities?

Remember... *"The master is committed to finding an opportunity for growth and improvement is every moment, every circumstance, every relationship, every task. Ideally, he seeks that opportunity regardless of his likes or dislikes, opinions or judgments about the circumstance, relationship or task."*

List three specific opportunities in your life right now for investing your attention and awareness:

- Identify one opportunity in your training as a master athlete
- Identify an opportunity in your occupation or field of study
- Identify a relationship with a family member or a close friend that merits a higher level of investment from you

Your choice to invest in each of these is *not* to obtain some desired result. That's just hoping for the future. (Recall the discussion on the Paradox of Control.) It is a choice to contribute more awareness and insight into your real-time engagement with each of these here and now.

When the old master is facing his opponent, there is one thing that is obviously absent in his demeanor. He is not angry with his opponent. He does not invest his precious awareness in judging his opponent. If you are earnest about bringing Kaizen to each of these opportunities in your life, you too must invest your precious attention in what is occurring here and now, and not in your judgments, desires, dislikes, etc. This is rigorous work!!

Action!!

Begin to use your endurance training sessions as a practice of investing your attention in each moment of the session. This can be difficult to do if you are fixated on a specific result from your session - like a desired pace. It can be done, but it requires rigorous work.

This is also true of investing our awareness and attention in a relationship. So many of our relationships get complicated and confusing when both parties are focused on specific (and often differing) results and not on what is really occurring in the moment between them.

Both in your training sessions and your interactions with others, it's OK to have goals. However it's essential that you invest your awareness and attention in what is occurring in the moment, free from any distraction or fixation on the results you want. This is a delicate balance! Your daily training session is a great opportunity to practice this balancing act. You may have specific goals you wish to achieve in your session. You can "hold" these goals as you invest your awareness and attention in each moment of your training by being conscious of each inhale and each exhale - *throughout your entire session.* Again, this is rigorous work!

Conscious Breathing

As master endurance athletes, this is easiest for us while swimming. In the water, *we have to be conscious of each breath. Our lives depend on it!* And our breath in swimming is not just for oxygen, it is also how we maintain buoyancy.

While cycling and running, you can synchronize your breath cycle with a specific number of pedal strokes or run strides for each inhale and each exhale. You can also begin to equate specific breath-stroke or breath-stride counts with your aerobic level.

For example, running with a:

- 3-stride inhale and 4-stride exhale may be an easy-moderate level.
- 2-stride inhale and 4-stride exhale may be a moderate level
- 2-stride inhale and 3-stride exhale may be a moderate-high level
- 2-stride inhale and 2-stride exhale is a high level

The mindful practice of conscious breathing has been around for *thousands of years*. It is the most ancient practice for investing our attention, of training our awareness and attention to stay in this moment.

It's Sensational!

In Chapter 1: The Fitness Cycle, we identified our neural system as the most responsive to endurance training. It's the system we focus on training for kaizen. Neural training develops our *kinetic intelligence* - the secret weapon that all those "over-the-hill" Ironman World Champions possess.

Neural training begins very simply: We fully invest our attention in the *sensations* that arise through our bodies with each stroke and stride of our training sessions.

Swim:

The most effective way to increase your speed in the water is to increase your hydrodynamics. Invest your attention to how the water flows along your body's skin surface:

- Begin with feeling that flow with your fingers, hand and forearm every time your hand enters and extends

- Feel that flow extending along your entire "vessel"

- Can you discern between resistance/drag and streamlining?

- Strive to feel your way through the water.

Bike:

Your bike is a prosthetic - an extension of your body. Invest your attention towards being able to feel that connection:

- Begin by feeling your connection to your bike through the saddle

- Can you remain quiet and still in the saddle as you pedal?

- Can you feel that you guide your bike mostly through this stable saddle connection?

- Observe your neck and shoulders

- Do you hold tension there?

Run:

While running is the most basic of all endurance sports, there's is a high risk of injury. To avoid injury, run further and recover faster, we must minimize the impact of each footfall:

- Feel every foot contact

- Where on the sole of your foot do you first feel contact with the ground?

- Is that initial contact different for your left versus your right?

- Look out at the horizon and observe how much vertical amplitude (bounce) you have with each stride: Less amplitude usually means less impact?

These are just a very few of literally thousands of sensations and combinations of sensations you can train your attention towards as you strive for the lifelong improvement of kinetic intelligence.

Chapter Summary

- Kaizen - lifelong improvement - occurs through our pursuit of mastery.

- Mastery arises when we are willing, prepared and able to welcome and embrace the challenges that arise in our lives as opportunities for growth and insight - even when we don't "like" them.

- There is no finish line to the lifelong improvement of our kaizen path.

- Mastery is not the same as control. We cannot control the circumstances or relationships of our lives. When we let go of our attempts to control, we have abundant energy and awareness to recognize and respond brilliantly to the opportunity that is arising.

- A master is committed to finding an opportunity for growth and improvement in every moment, every circumstance, every relationship, every task. She is able to detach from her likes or dislikes, opinions or judgments, desires, fears, etc.

- The master relentlessly strives to accurately perceive what is occurring in the present moment.

- Mastery requires that we fully invest our attention Here and Now.

- As Helen Keller showed us, there are no limits to our ability to perceive or to express. Our experience-ability is infinite.

- Our infinite experience-ability exists only in the present moment. Our pursuit of mastery cannot occur in the past or in the future. It requires rigorous training for us to really Be Here Now.

- As kaizen athletes, we have the opportunity to train and develop the essential skills necessary to fully invest our attention and awareness in this moment and to enjoy lifelong improvement. These essential skills are called "mindfulness skills". We can develop these mindfulness skills at the same time we are training as endurance athletes.

CHAPTER FOUR:
SHARPEN YOUR AXE

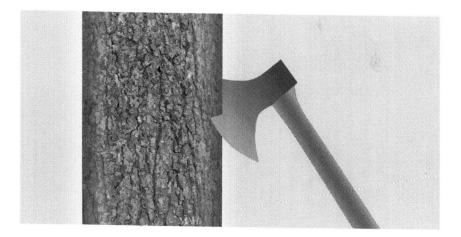

"Give me six hours to chop down a tree, and I will spend the first four hours sharpening the axe." - Abe Lincoln

Introduction

Imagine trying to chop down a tree with a sledge hammer instead of an axe: Elite-level aerobic fitness combined with monstrous muscular strength will not help you cut through more wood with that sledge hammer. It's well worth the investment of time and energy to select the correct tool and prepare it well before taking on the task.

As master athletes, we need to sharpen our "endurance axes" before we launch from the starting line of the race. It takes more than great aerobic fitness and muscular strength to perform well, and to actually *enjoy* the challenge. That endurance axe we sharpen is our kinetic intelligence. With kinetic intelligence, we cut a precise and clean incision - from the starting line to the finish line. Every efficient stroke, every efficient stride is part of that incision.

We hone kinetic intelligence by training neural fitness. How fortunate for us that we can continue to build this neural fitness for decades beyond aerobic prime! There are no walls to stop us.

In this chapter, we explore the process of sharpening our endurance axe so we can successfully pursue kinetic intelligence. We begin that exploration with a paradigm shift in how we approach training and racing. But first…

The Countdown

"*Three!*" World Champions win races with high levels of kinetic intelligence.

"*Two!*" We acquire kinetic intelligence as we increase and improve neural fitness.

"*One!*" We gain neural fitness when we *approach* each training session with a 100% investment of our awareness and attention.

"*Go!*" With that 100% investment, we maximize the return on our training investment - race day, and every day.

So, how do we approach each training session with a really sharp axe? How do we arrive at the starting line of the race - indeed, at the start of each and every training session - with that 100% investment of our awareness and attention?

Let's begin by exploring a new way to view our training sessions and our races.

Eyes On the Prize

As athletes, we are goal-driven. We've got our eyes on the prize. This drive to achieve our goal gives us that day-to-day discipline and perseverance to get out the door and complete the workout. In the shower, after the finish of the session, we check off another step to finish line. Not only are we training our skills as endurance athletes, we are developing healthy life skills as well - like the abilities to follow through and to persevere, even when things get tough. However...

This goal-drive can also get us into trouble. We are often prone to ignore warning signs from our bodies that we are not balancing the stress of training with adequate recovery and adaptation. We treat our training program like a holy scripture. *"This is the step-by-step guide that's guaranteed to get me to that finish line glory. I have to follow it to the number."*

Come race day, with our eager eyes fixed on that prize, when the cannon booms, we often launch off the starting line as if the finish line was just a hundred meters away. This can have devastating consequences in that long day ahead.

The strong fixation to achieve our goals can also get us into trouble outside athletics: With our eyes on that prize, we often fail to *listen accurately* to what others are communicating to us. Our determination to "make the sale" or to get the result can result in miscommunications and misunderstandings that result in conflict. This can lead to long-term resentment and - in the case of a marriage - even divorce.

Or, with that fixation, we may lack patience to complete an ordinary task well, because we are in a hurry to check it off the list and stamp it *"Mission Accomplished!"*

Athlete Or...?

Here's a typical athlete scenario. Joe Primetime wants to do Lake Placid Ironman next summer. Joe hires a coach and declares, *"Coach, I don't care what it takes! Just get me to that finish line! I want to hear Mike Reilly say 'Joe Primetime, you are an IRONMAN!!'"* With a locked-and-loaded focus on the result, Joe is going to follow (and maybe exceed) his coach's step-by-step plan - come hell or high water.

Now let's look at a different scenario - an *artist* scenario: An aspiring musician begins to study violin. When she seeks out her teacher she doesn't declare *"Coach, I want to play First Violin for Beethoven's Fifth Symphony at the JFK Symphony Hall next year! I don't care what it takes, just get me there!"*

The musician doesn't chase a Big Goal. Instead, she patiently develops her *craft* as a musician. She focuses on cultivating excellent technique, on crafting a desirable and distinctive "voice". This voice will enable her to play with excellence, and not just speed. And that *patiently crafted* voice will bring the opportunities to play in fine symphony halls, and an enduring, satisfying career.

Miraculously, Joe Primetime makes it to the shoreline of Mirror Lake for the start of Lake Placid Ironman - despite a few episodes of overtraining and a nagging achilles tendon. He dives in and begins the 2-loop swim, going out too fast for the first half-mile. When the weariness sets into his arms and lungs, he slows down.

On the 2-loop bike course, Joe doesn't need the 5-Mile Markers. He closely monitors his GPS unit, counting down the miles even though he misses the incredible scenery of the course. By the second loop he can feel it in his legs. He tries to ignore the fatigue and focus on the mileage countdown. When he finally dismounts in the transition zone, his legs are despondent. It's like learning how to walk again. Like the swim, Joe was a little too eager on the bike.

Primetime spends 15 minutes in transition, a little panicked about his condition. He assures himself over and over, *"I can do this. Just 26.2 miles to go."* Once out of transition, again he sets his tunnel vision on the mileage countdown. During his months of training, he felt so confident about his running. Now, he is reduced to walking the miles. But all he has to do is keeping counting down, counting down... Until he finally reaches the bright lights of the finish line, and Mike Reilly's booming voice.

Now, let's return to the musician. After years of patient and diligent practice - both alone and in ensembles - she is able to sing as naturally and fluently with her violin as she speaks with her own voice. Her violin is now part of her being. She is invited to play First Violin for Beethoven's Fifth Symphony. As the conductor cues the symphony, she invests her full awareness and attention to craft *each note* she plays - giving each the space and time and richness it needs. She is not counting down how many more bars of music she must play until the end. Instead, she is present with each perfect note and how it fits with the entire symphony.

Focus On This Stride

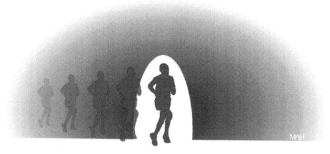

Simple Advice

For those of us who are striving to finish that first iron distance triathlon, or to finally finish one without misery and pain, I offer this advice: Ironman is not one-hundred-and-forty-point-six-miles. It is *one mile*... one hundred and forty point six times.

Here is the secret to going the distance, especially a distance that is longer than you have ever finished before: Craft the first stroke, the first stride perfectly. And then, craft the next stoke, the next stride perfectly. And then...

To craft each stroke, each stride perfectly, use your kinetic intelligence, rather than fixating on how far you have left to go, or what your pace or power output should be. Invest all of your attention and awareness in *this stroke, this stride*.

Be an artist with your craft, as well as an athlete with your goals.

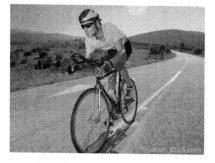
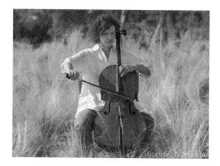

Athlete:

Result-focused: Clearly defined goal (race/event): Distance, terrain, time, format

Quantity (metrics)-driven: Measures progress: Pace/speed, distance, heart rate, power output

Artist:

Process-focused: Craft each note, each brush stroke perfectly

Quality-driven: Pitch, timbre, duration of note; hue, color, texture, thickness of brush stroke

Master Athlete/Artist:

Focuses on process to patiently approach goal

Achieves goal through well-crafted strokes/strides,

Chooses pace in each moment appropriate to internal and external circumstances rather than some plan hatched at the desk months ago

Approach: Sharpening the Kaizen-durance Axe

As master athletes, how can we balance the motivation of our goal drive with the lifelong craft of kinetic intelligence? How can we begin each session and each race with a full investment of our awareness and attention in the present moment, while we patiently and gracefully approach our goals? Quite simply...

We begin at the beginning. Or maybe we begin *before* the beginning: We begin by sharpening the Kaizen durance Axe. It's all in our *approach*.

As master athletes, our training sessions begin *before* the first stroke or stride. First we summon the awareness and attention to engage kinetic intelligence. We do this during the *approach* leading up to that first stroke or stride.

Again, picture the wise old master. As he faces his opponent, he clears his mind and relaxes his body to prepare. Together, his patient, clear mind and relaxed, supple, alert body become his sharp axe. As a master, he uses the power of the Beginner's Mind.

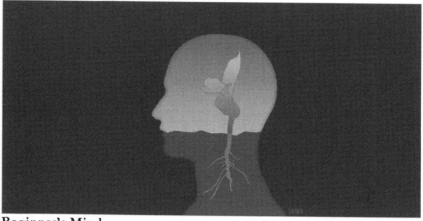

Beginner's Mind

"In the mind of the Beginner, there are infinite possibilities. In the mind of the Expert, there are very few."

With Beginner's Mind, we approach each session, each race as a new experience, with a unique set of circumstances - both internal (self) and external (environment). We approach with the heightened awareness and fresh curiosity of the Beginner. We are primed to explore, discover and learn something new each time. Beginner's Mind accelerates our acquisition of kinetic intelligence.

The Expert approaches with just one result in the crosshairs of the scope - ignoring all else. In our goal-driven mode, that result usually mandates a specific level of metabolic intensity for a specific duration. There is no allowance or flexibility for learning and discovery. Many "numbers-driven" athletes have little awareness for what is occurring in the moment beyond what the heart rate monitor, power meter or GPS displays. (This frequently means their technique is poor.)

Beginner's Mind is not "Naive Mind" or "Ignorant Mind". The wise old master embodies decades of experience and training when he faces his opponent. However, with Beginner's Mind, he remains open and alert to any possible circumstance that may arise. This openness imbues him with the suppleness, flexibility, creativity and rapid response of a child.

As master athletes, we too approach each session, each race with the wisdom of our extensive past experience. However, we fully engage our awareness and attention in the uniqueness of the present moment. We accurately perceive what is occurring and arising within us and around us here and now. Each stroke and each stride is crafted from a balance of our accumulated past experience and the myriad conditions that are arising in the present moment.

To put it simply: Not one of us has ever lived through *this present moment* before. We all arrive in this moment as Beginners. Cultivating and engaging Beginner's Mind is a most essential part of our approach as master athletes so that we can gain the most out each training session and each race.

Sharpen Your Axe: Beginner's Mind

To approach each training session with Beginner's Mind, arrive at the start of your session - even the most mundane - with the curiosity of a child:

- Pause before you begin

- Close your eyes and breathe deeply a few times as you clear your mind and relax your body

- As you pause, pretend this is the first time you have ever ridden your bike, or jumped in the pool, or…

- Welcome the infinite possibility for discovery in this training session. After all, there are no limits to your experience-ability

- What is unique in your experience of beginning today?

Sharpen Your Axe: Finalist's Mind

You can also approach each session with *Finalist's Mind*. Can you recall a time when you were sick or injured, and unable to train or race? Do you remember your resolve at that time to really savor every moment of your athletic life when you could resume your passion? Along with the curiosity of the child, arrive at the start of your session with the patience and gratitude of someone who has just been granted one more day to live:

- Again, pause before you begin. Breathe, clear your mind and relax your body

- Pretend this will be the last time ever in your life that you will have the opportunity to ride your bike, swim in the pool, or…

- Feel gratitude for the health and ability you have, for the opportunity that lies right here in front of you here and now

- Pique your senses so you are aware and will remember every moment of your session

- Approach your session as if your life depends on it: Imagine the high risk of the martial artist

When we engage both Beginner's Mind and Finalist's Mind, we invest more of our infinite experience-ability in each and every training session. It's as if there is no past, and no future. In each session, with a sharp axe, we have the opportunity to increase that rich resource of neural fitness.

We maximize return on our aerobic investment by generously investing our most abundant resources in each moment - our awareness and attention.

Sharpen Your Axe: The Golden Opportunity

Your *recovery sessions* are the golden opportunity to practice and master the Kaizen-durance Approach:

- Even if you normally train with other athletes, conduct some of your recovery sessions in solitude

- Leave the heart rate monitor, power meter and GPS units at home. To practice honing your approach, you need to let go of staring at a screen and "hitting the numbers" so you can really sense what is actually occurring in that intelligent instrument called "your body". (The exceptions: A watch to log the time of your session, a heart rate monitor if you have a tendency to train too hard on your recovery days)

- Allow at least five minutes of your actual training time just to pause and conjure your Beginner's Mind and/or Finalist's Mind: to sharpen your axe: This means you are crediting yourself with training time for just practicing stillness both mentally and physically

- Choose a quiet location, close your eyes, and let your body be still (either standing, sitting or lying down)

- Pause to breathe and calm your mind: For at least ten breath cycles, really feel each inhale and each exhale

- Allow the "hurry-up-and-get-going urge" to rise up if it does: Observe it. What body sensations do you feel in this urge? What thoughts and/or feelings do you have with it? Let the urge go.

- Reassure yourself that you are sharpening your axe in preparation: Honing your ability to craft every stroke or stride perfectly, to cut that clean incision to the finish line

- Picture the wise old martial artist: patient, calm, slow, deliberate, confident, graceful - even in the midst of chaos

- What are you grateful for right now?

- Open your eyes and look around, really seeing what is around you

As you begin your recovery session:

- Be conscious of each breath from start to finish (This alone is a challenging task)

- With that breath consciousness, begin your session very slowly, striving to keep your breathing slow and deep, your body relaxed, your mind clear and alert (Remember, this is a recovery session)

- Craft each stroke, each stride with the grace and ease of the wise old martial arts master

- Synchronize your breath with your strokes/strides (Running example: inhale 3 strides, exhale 4 strides)

- Give yourself permission to move slowly

- Explore specific body sensations as you begin to glide forward

- Through those body sensations, and the relationships between those sensations, strive to discover or experience something new in your stroke or stride

- Right from the start, closely monitor your Rate of Perceived Exertion (RPE): Sense what actually happens within your body as your aerobic level slowly increases - in the muscles, through your respiration and circulatory system

- During your recovery session, keep your RPE at or below 4 or 5 on a scale of 1-10

- Play with your form and technique. Seek out a feeling of grace and ease, a sense of flow

- Look for tensions in your body and use your conscious breath and feeling of ease and grace to dissolve the tensions - even if you have to slow down.

Rate Of Perceived Exertion

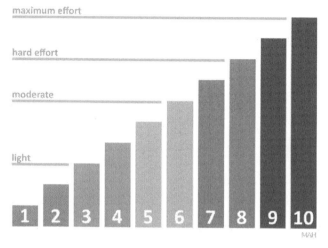

Quality Assurance

Our *approach* to every activity and in every relationship has a profound bearing on the quality of our experience. While we may not *control* outright the result, our approach determines what resources and assets we show up with. The most valuable asset we can bring to any activity or relationship is our infinite experience-ability. That begins when we generously invest our awareness and attention to optimize our perceptive acuity. We make that investment as we craft our approach.

We have the opportunity each time we train for endurance to also train our approach. We just explored some ways to strengthen our approaching skills. When you complete your training session, pause to evaluate your *experience:*

- How aware were you with each breath?

- How much awareness did you invest in each stroke or stride?

- With your Beginner's Mind, what did you discover during your training today?

- With your Finalist's Mind, what are you grateful for in your training today?

- What skills and attributes - physical and/or mental - did you build today?

- Can you approach other areas of your life today with those skills and attributes?

What can we do if we feel that we did not summon our awareness and invest our attention, if we failed to craft an effective approach? We can do the same thing that we do when we succeed or even excel in our approach: We learn and grow. We will certainly have judgments of "good" or "bad", but praising ourselves, or beating up on ourselves will not help either way. This is a great opportunity to be patient and to persevere.

Chapter Summary

Kinetic intelligence is our strongest asset as master athletes. When we approach each training session with our full awareness and attention, we consistently grow that intelligence and the return on our investment of time and energy. Approach is the process of summoning our full awareness and attention to the task that awaits us.

We develop and train effective "approach skills" by cultivating qualities of mindfulness such as patience, curiosity and gratitude. (We explore and investigate extensively the skills of mindfulness in Book 3.)

Our focus on a specific athletic goal (like a desired race performance) can provide motivation, discipline and perseverance in the months of preparation. However, that same drive to achieve can distract us from what is actually occurring in the present moments of our training sessions. We may get ahead of ourselves. In endurance training and racing, this can result in poor pacing, inefficient technique, even injury. It can also be detrimental in other areas of our lives, particularly our relationships with others.

Compared to athletes, artists are typically more *process*-focused, rather than goal-focused. Process focus emphasizes the diligent acquisition of skills and the patient development of a craft. Balancing our athletic goals with an artistic appreciation for and commitment to the skills and craft of kaizen-durance can inspire us to be more deliberate in our approach.

Two effective tools that empower our approach are Beginner's Mind and Finalist's Mind.

With Beginner's Mind, we approach each training session, each experience in life with the heightened awareness and fresh curiosity of the Beginner. We are primed to explore, discover and experience something new each time. Beginner's Mind accelerates our acquisition of kinetic intelligence.

With Finalist's Mind, we approach each session, each experience in life as if it is our last: There is no guarantee we will achieve that goal we have in the future. We are patient and grateful for the opportunity this moment holds for us right now. Finalist's Mind also accelerates our acquisition of kinetic intelligence.

When we combine Beginner's Mind and Finalist's Mind, we relinquish our attachment to the past and to the future. We are able to fully invest our awareness and attention in the present moment. We show up with a very sharp axe.

Recovery sessions are golden opportunities to sharpen our perceptive acuity through an effective approach. Begin these sessions by allotting five-to-ten minutes just to focus on sharpening your axe. Leave all of the monitors and meters at home. During your approach and your actual training, be aware of each breath.

Begin your session very slowly. Throughout the session:

- Craft each stroke, each stride with the grace and ease of the wise old martial arts master

- Synchronize each breath with your strokes and strides

- Explore the sensations that arise, and the myriad relationships between those sensations

- Right from the start, closely monitor your Rate of Perceived Exertion (RPE). You can quantify it on a scale of 1-10

- Keep your RPE at or below 4-5

During your recovery session, you don't have any quantifiable goals to achieve. Instead, when you finish your session, evaluate the *quality* of your experience based on how aware and attentive you were throughout the session, and the skills and attributes you developed.

Finally, consider this: The study of fighting skills is known as Martial *Arts,* not Martial Sports. Like expressive artists (musicians, painters, dancers, etc.) martial artists appreciate patient and diligent practice and the commitment to lifelong improvement. Their's is a pursuit of mastery through perceptive acuity and infinite experience-ability.

What's Next?

OK! We have paused to craft our approach. It's time to train, to practice!!

In the next chapter, we finally get to explore the real "stuff" of our craft as master endurance athletes. We will identify and explore specific skills we can pursue and develop during our training sessions to hone the individual craft that makes us each a unique master endurance athlete.

CHAPTER FIVE:
KINETIC INTELLIGENCE:
WISDOM OF THE MASTER ATHLETE

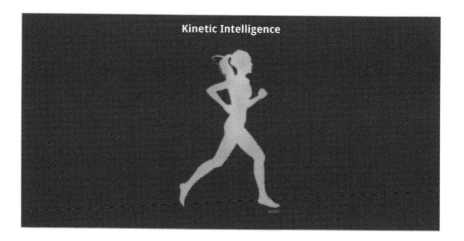

Introduction

I coined the term "*kinetic intelligence*" during my collegiate study of modern dance, as I began to discover and activate regions of my brain and body that empowered me to move my body with more precision, ease and grace. My formal study of kinetic intelligence still continues four decades later through my daily kaizen practice of endurance athletics.

In this chapter, we identify and explore kinetic intelligence and how to pursue it so that we can go far beyond what we thought possible as master athletes. We begin with a working definition:

Kinetic intelligence is the skill to occupy and animate our bodies with precision, grace and ease. It includes:

- The ability to clearly perceive how we are moving right now

- The skill to "problem-solve" so that we can adapt and refine our movements

- The ability to clearly imprint and reliably recall these new, wiser movements

So, how do we cultivate kinetic intelligence? Let's start with some sage advise offered of the Kung Fu TV series by the blind old master.

"Ah! Patience grasshopper, patience."

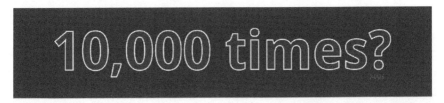

Patience

In the film "Karate Kid", we are first introduced to the wise old master (Mr. Miyagi) in a peculiar way: Young Daniel enters the maintenance shop to report a plumbing problem in the apartment he and his mother have just moved into. We see an old man from behind, in a cluttered workshop, sitting in a chair at his desk. He is holding chopsticks in his hand, snapping at the air as he tries in vain to catch a fly that is buzzing around.

Our first impression is that perhaps this old guy is a bit crazy. After all, who would waste so much time attempting to catch a fly with chopsticks? Why not use a fly swatter and be done with it?

Later in the film, Daniel convinces Mr. Miyagi to teach him Karate so that he can face the bullies in school who are making his life miserable. Full of enthusiasm, Daniel shows up at Mr. Miyagi's house early one day for his first fighting lesson. Much to his dismay, Mr. Miyagi hands him a tin of old-fashioned paste wax and instructs young Daniel to wax one of his classic old cars. His instructions - perhaps the most memorable line from the film: "*Wax on with right hand. Wax off with left hand.*" He demonstrates the correct circular motion for each hand and walks away.

Daniel proceeds to wax the classic car - with a few more directives about the correct circular motion for applying and buffing. Mr. Miyagi also instructs him to "*Breathe in through nose. Breathe out through mouth.*" Hours later, when he has finished, he reports back to Mr. Miyagi, with great pride. Mr. Miyagi takes him to the next car. ...There are perhaps eight cars.

Days later, Daniel finishes waxing the last car. "*Surely now I have earned my first fighting lesson.*" Instead, Mr Miyagi instructs Daniel to sand the spacious deck surrounding Mr. Miyagi's house - again using specific hand movements. And then, after the deck, Daniel must paint the fence that surrounds the entire compound. "*Big boards right hand. Small boards left hand.*" ...Both sides of the fence. "*Breathe in through nose, out through mouth.*"

Eventually, feeling he has been conned, Daniel finally loses his patience and his temper. It is only then that Mr. Miyagi shows him that the specific buffing, sanding and painting movements have trained him for the specific hand and arm movements that will make him an effective fighter. Before Daniel can strive for his goal, he must patiently develop the craft through countless repetitions.

There is an adage about developing and mastering a skill - specifically a movement skill. To do it well, one must practice *ten thousand* times. Repetition is essential in the pursuit of mastery, yes. However, the required number of repetitions is not dead set at ten thousand. It may take far more; it may take far fewer.

(Note: This is often called "*muscle memory*". We explore this in more depth in Book 2.)

Practice does not make perfect. (Practice makes *permanent*.) *Perfect* practice makes perfect. With a deliberate, patient and mindful approach, and a very sharp axe of perceptive acuity, our practice is ever closer to perfection from the very first repetition. No longer will it take ten thousand repetitions.

Kinetic intelligence is the *wisdom* we acquire as master athletes. Wisdom distills from decades of experience. To cultivate and acquire wisdom requires patience and perseverance. We value wisdom if we have a clear vision of the benefits it provides. Then we are willing to patiently invest the time and energy in training for that wisdom.

As master athletes, we approach daily endurance training patiently - less attached to short term goals, and more appreciative of the *process* that leads to kinetic intelligence.

Revisiting the Paradox of Control

Recalling the image of the wise old sage: A brash young warrior begins to attack. The old sage calmly responds with easy efficient movements. He does not try to control or dominate his opponent. Instead, he taps into the forces that are already "at play" - forces that are provided by his opponent. Even when he is fighting to defend his life, he appears to be in balance and harmony. He embodies effortless power.

The Master's effortless power arises from the "Paradox of Control": He has a clear vision of his goal - to disarm and pacify his opponent. But he is not fixated on the result he desires. Such attachment to his desired outcome, and the haste and impatience to get to his result would cloud his perceptive acuity. In his feeble old age, it is this well-trained, sharp perceptive acuity that is his greatest weapon - one far more powerful than the robust strength and exuberant vigor of youth.

Our Sensei has patiently, over the decades, sharpened the axe of his perceptive acuity so that he can easily, efficiently and effortlessly cut down even the mightiest tree with very few strokes. If his perceptions were dull - like his younger, inexperienced opponent, he would struggle to fell that great tree, as if with a maul: Even the heaviest blows with the biggest maul won't cut through the tree.

The Master transforms his opponent from a formidable foe set on inflicting harm into a resource of energy and forces that aide the Master in achieving his goal. He does this using his kinetic intelligence, rather than brute strength. He embraces the Paradox of Control:

- He cannot control the intent or the actions his opponent

- Yet, he can choose to embrace his opponent's intent and actions and re-orchestrate them towards his desired outcome

Embracing the Paradox of Control:

We do not waste energy trying to control the thoughts, intents and actions of others, or the events that are arising.

We do not waste energy judging the thoughts, intents and actions of others or the events that are arising.

Instead, without resistance, we choose to embrace what is arising exactly as it is and to seize the opportunities that are arising through these events.

We cannot control the world around us. However, we have the opportunity to choose our response:

- We can choose not to resist and fight

- We can choose to embrace, accommodate and blend with what is arising

As we re-orchestrate the forces and circumstances that are arising, it appears as if we are in control. This is the paradox. We solve this paradox through the power of our *choice*.

The P.A.G.E.S. Movements

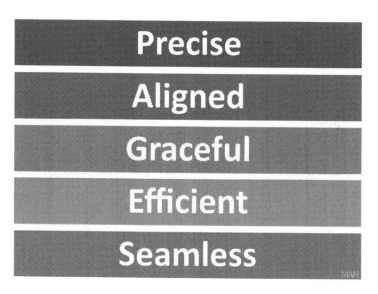

The Essence of Kinetic Intelligence: P.A.G.E.S. Movements

With perceptive acuity and patient training, the Sensei responds to his opponent brilliantly with "P.A.G.E.S." movements:

- Precise

- Aligned

- Graceful

- Efficient

- Seamless

Through PAGES movements, the Sensei wields his effortless power. We will explore each of these qualities in a moment, and how they pertain to endurance sports. But first, let's return briefly to patience, ten thousand reps and...

Neural Plasticity

Developing PAGES movements may well require decades of patience and perseverance, practicing the same movements over and over again. But even the small steps of improvement you make each day, each week will translate into kaizen. Kaizen happens just like it did for the Karate Kid: "*Wax on right hand. Wax off left hand.*"

In my experience facilitating thousands of people in their pursuit of swimming efficiency, the determining factor for how rapidly someone can improve is known in scientific circles as *neural plasticity*.

Remember, our neural system is the system that responds and improves the most to athletic training. This is due to neural *plasticity* - essentially the neural system's ability to learn. Our metabolic and muscular systems, are almost entirely "physical", with limited potential to actually *learn*. However, our neural system - as an interface between body and brain - is quite capable of learning. Regardless of your age, your neural system has a seemingly infinite capacity to learn and improve - a capacity that does not diminish until very late in life if you keep it healthy and challenge it wisely through the Fitness Cycle.

We don't need to bang our heads against the Aerobic Wall as we experience the slow decline of metabolic fitness. Yes, we may be losing aerobic capacity, but through kinetic intelligence, we discover how to move with less aerobic capacity. Your only chance to preserve your performance is to change the way you train - through neural fitness and kinetic intelligence.

If we approach our athletic training, and our pursuit of PAGES movements with the sharp axe of perceptive acuity, we are priming our neural system to maximally respond and adapt to our training. The "*perfect*" in perfect practice requires perceptive acuity. With this, we train PAGES movements at our highest potential. We maximize return on our aerobic investment.

Hence my relentless emphasis on our approach. And now, with a very sharp axe...

Kinetic Intelligence: The Master Athlete's Weapon

Like the old sage who uses his kinetic intelligence to easily disarm and pacify his opponent, we too use kinetic intelligence to defy the conventions of age as master endurance athletes. With kinetic intelligence, we are able to:

- Move forward faster and/or further

- Use less energy

- Decrease our risk of injury

- Increase our rate of recovery

On our kaizen-durance path, we can *enjoy* that pursuit, and experience success and satisfaction regardless of whether we achieve our goals.

As master athletes, the expression of kinetic intelligence arises in our PAGES strokes and strides.

Introduction PAGES Movements

I have chosen "PAGES" as an easy-to-remember acronym for these 5 qualities. However, in my experience, we build and sequence these qualities in a slightly different order. That is, we begin with one of these qualities - "Aligned" - as the first in the sequence. Alignment is required for the next quality - Precision - and so forth. That building sequence is:

- Aligned

- Precise

- Seamless

- Efficient

- Graceful

This sequence is not a "one-time" deal: While we first focus on crafting alignment in our movements before striving for precision, we will continue to pursue alignment - the most profound of these qualities - for the rest of our lives. We don't ever really "finish being aligned". And we actually pursue and craft all of these qualities simultaneously. As we explore each, this sequence will be more apparent. So let's begin with…

Aligned

Alignment is the first element of PAGES movements - the foundational element. In our bodies, that "foundation" is our skeletal structure - with it's *three hundred and sixty* joints. Unlike most conventional rigid and fixed structures, our bones and joints comprise an *articulate and interactive* structure.

The pelvis and spine serve as the very core of this complex structure. The spine is comprised 34 vertebrae joined together by 33 joints that are flexible in every plane of movement, as well as rotation. Our spine provides structure for the torso, as well as our shoulders, neck and head. Since the main trunk of nerves - known as the the spinal cord - passes through the vertebrae and joints - to interface brain and body - neural function of every part of the body, including arms and legs, hands and feet, is affected - either positively or adversely - by the alignment or misalignment of our vertebral joints.

The pelvis is an assembly of bones shaped like a big "half-bowl", closed in the back, open in the front. The spine connects to the pelvis along the sides of the sacral vertebrae. These connection sites are known collectively as the "sacroiliac" or "S.I." joints - with one on each (left and right) side of the vertebrae. In addition to the SI joints, our hip joints are also integral to the pelvis. This means that the pelvis unites *upper and lower body together.*

For every swim stroke, pedal stroke, run stride, etc., the *pelvic core* serves as the:

- Center of gravity

- Center and source of movement

- Union of upper and lower body

The fore-aft tilt of the pelvis - known as "*pelvic pitch*" - is critical for aligning and integrating the upper and lower halves of the body. Pelvic pitch also affects our ability to engage and use the powerful pelvic core muscles to produce strong and efficient strokes and strides. Hence pelvic pitch and spine alignment are the very foundation of every movement.

While pelvic pitch and spine alignment are complex enough, we also strive for alignment of the bones in the extremities:

- Through the hip, knee and ankle joints, we align the bones of our upper and lower legs, and our feet

- Through the shoulder, elbow and wrist joints, we align the bones of our upper and lower arms and our hands

As we swim, pedal and run, our extremities must swing, flex and extend in the plane of our direction of travel:

- In the water, alignment minimizes drag in the water - the most significant determinant of swimming efficiency. (Consider that novice swimmers are 1-3% efficient, while world-class swimmers are 9-10% efficient. Improving efficiency by a single percent can result in significant improvement in performance. Efficiency begins with alignment.)

- In cycling, we align the hip, knee, ankle and foot so that all the energy of each pedal stroke moves us forward and not side-to-side. Side-to-side deviations here make us unstable on the bike and increase our risk of injury.

- In running, we align both the legs and arms to swing in the direction of travel. Similar to cycling, any lateral deviations waste energy and may cause injury.

With *three hundred and sixty* joints to monitor and align, its easy to see just how essential awareness, attention and neural training are.

…And that's just the start. When we consider alignment, we must consider a fundamental force we are aligning *with*. Alignment with this force is even more essential than aligning with our direction of travel. This force provides us with feedback and orientation for alignment: When we "listen" to this force, alignment becomes clear. We will deeply consider and explore this fundamental force, this vital source of orientation in the next chapter. For now, we let's move on to…

Precise

I have watched several times a video of the late Bruce Lee playing Ping Pong with two expert players. They are playing together, as a team, on one side of the table, using Ping Pong paddles. Bruce Lee, playing solo, is not using a Ping Pong paddle. Instead, he is using *nunchucks* - clearly a disadvantage. Yet, with incredible precision, he never misses a shot and is able to win each volley. The precision of his movements is astounding.

By comparison, the precision of a single pedal stroke or run stride seems quite simple. Yet, when we consider the biomechanics of a swim stroke, pedal stroke or run stride, there are innumerable elements.

Let's consider a pedal stroke, perhaps the simplest of the three: Pedal stroke precision is comprised of:

- Pelvic pitch and low back profile to maximize pelvic core muscle engagement for stability and power

- Alignment of hips, knees, ankles and feet through pedal stroke

- Relationship of joint angles at all phases of the stroke cycle

- Synchronicity/timing of various joint articulations (especially ankle articulation and foot angle on pedal) during all phases of pedal stroke

- Optimal combination of cadence and "stroke length" (determined on the bike by gear choice)

- Amount of force applied to each pedal at each degree of pedal rotation

…And this is just a simple pedal stroke!

Just as there is no one perfect swim stroke, or one perfect run stride, there is no one perfect pedal stroke that all cyclists should aspire to. Why? There are infinite variations between each of us, such as:

- Different proportional lengths of femur (upper leg) vs. fibula/tibia (lower leg), and foot length

- Varying ranges of motion for each individual's left and right hip, knee and ankle

- Varying ranges of stability for each individual's left and right hip, knee, ankle joints and the many joints of each foot

- Varying neural function for each individual's left and right sides

- Varying degrees of strength for individual's left and right legs

- Varying degrees of aerobic capacity

Precise movements also respond to myriad environmental factors, such as the terrain (hills in cycling and running, chop in open water swimming). Variations in response to these include adjustments to alignment, stroke/stride length (which changes all the joint angles through all phases of each) and cadence.

Precise strokes and strides are intentional, controlled and coordinated. Both alignment and precision require stability, mobility and agility - collectively known as "functional strength". Functional strength requires a lot more than well-toned major muscles. There are hundreds of small muscles and connective tissues that are essential to precise movements. And all of these must be guided and coordinated by an "intelligent" neural system.

Without precision, our strokes and strides fail to respond to the ever-changing environment that requires a unique and… well, *precise* response for each. When our movements are precise, we:

- Use less energy

- Transfer energy efficiently through the body

- Greatly reduce the risk of injury

With precision, we gain these advantages not only when the terrain and environmental factors are ideal, but also when they are challenging. We can adjust each stroke, each stride.

System Overload?

So far, we have considered just the first two elements of PAGES movements. The complexity of each of these alone seems overwhelming. How can we possibly monitor and control so many things at one time? This is simply overwhelming to our "linear-mode" part of the brain.

This "linear mode" is the part of the brain that is reading the words on this page. It's the part we most inhabit and engage in our day-to-day interactions. (As I say, "we like to reside in the penthouse suite of the frontal cortex".) However, this frontal cortex is *not* the part of the brain that teams up with our body for movement. We cannot generate movements of any kind using only the frontal cortex and its linear processors. For that, we must engage other regions of the brain - regions we consider to be *lower* than that penthouse suite.

(Note: A neuroanatomist would dispute the specific terms I am using to identify these various regions of the brain - linear mode, frontal cortex. However, it's important to note that we consciously inhabit the linear language regions of the brain far more than other regions, like those that coordinate and process spacial tasks such as movement. We explore this more in Book 2.)

For now, we must trust that there are other intelligence centers in the brain that are quite capable of teaming up with the body via the neural system to craft brilliant PAGES movements. Each of us began tapping into those "movement centers" of the brain in infancy - using our arms and hands to bring food (and most everything else) to our mouths, and then learning to balance, stand and walk.

Actually, we constantly engage these areas of the brain throughout our daily activities. It's just that we are not so conscious of these intelligence centers as we are of that penthouse suite of the frontal cortex. (Verbal and written language are the primary means of transaction in our daily lives.) However, these are the parts of the brain we rigorously activate *and exercise* as we acquire the kinetic intelligence of the master athlete.

Although he was not directly conscious of it, young Daniel was developing the kinetic intelligence required for karate as he waxed all those cars and painted that entire fence. And, each of those movements - buffing, sanding, painting - was...

Seamless

Our movements need to be seamless - that is continuous, flowing, often circular. It's easy to see how essential this quality is in our swim strokes, pedal strokes and running strides. If our strides and strokes are choppy and abrupt, we are constantly breaking the momentum.

With choppy and abrupt movements, we are constantly accelerating and decelerating. It requires lots of energy to change velocity, to start and stop - precious energy that is not actually moving us forward. Abrupt and choppy movements also increase our risk of injury significantly.

An example of a not-seamless movement: A long, leaping running stride with a heavy, hard heel strike and lots of up-and-down vertical amplitude. Running biomechanics experts have studied the form and technique of various runners, including elite marathoners. The fastest runners spend less time on the ground and have very little up-and-down bobbing as they run.

I have seen calculations that show that a rise and fall of 12 inches for every stride in a marathon is like adding a stair-climbing ascent and descent of the Empire State Building. That makes for a lot more "hills" over that 26.2 miles!! (Way more effort and energy.) And a lot more impact with every foot strike. (Increased stress and increased risk of injury.)

The difference between the elite 2:07 marathoner and you or me? For sure there is an aerobic difference. Even with dedicated and consistent metabolic training, we probably won't even get close in that realm. However, we can certainly improve on the seamless quality of each run stride - minimizing the time our feet are actually on the ground, and running forward, instead of up and down. These are the qualities of an elite runner that we can all aspire to.

Seamless strides and strokes maintain a constant flowing movement with an even velocity and momentum. Can you guess what seamless strokes and strides require? Yup, alignment and precision. Put all three of them together, and we are now knocking at the door of...

Efficient

In the context of endurance sports, efficiency is a measure of our ability to move forward with less energy and effort. Benefits may include:

- Increased speed (go faster)

- Increased endurance (go farther)

- Increased rate of recovery (faster progression through the fitness cycle)

- Decreased risk of injury (less pain and damage)

- Increased enjoyment when training and racing (more motivation)

Efficiency is perhaps the "Holy Grail" of endurance sports. It is a lifetime pursuit: There is always an opportunity to increase efficiency, no matter what our age. And that's great news!! Efficiency is a significant element of kaizen for master athletes.

Efficiency begins with our ability to generate our strokes and strides from the "stable platform" of the pelvic core. We maximize the use of these largest, strongest and most enduring muscles of the body that are closest to both our oxygen and energy supply chains.

All of the elements presented so far in this chapter are essential to efficiency: Efficiency requires that our strokes/strides are aligned, precise and seamless.

Finally, like the effortless power expressed in the efficient moves of the martial arts Sensei, we maximize efficiency when we draw upon and orchestrate forces available to us and minimize our own force generation. In the next chapter, we will explore the most powerful natural force on Earth - a force that each of us has continuous access to.

Before we begin that exploration, let's consider the last element of our PAGES strokes and strides...

Graceful

As an element of PAGES movements, grace may be the least measurable and most subjective of the five. In my experience, grace is the overall synergy of the other four elements. We can see *grace* in the way the wise old Sensei responds to his opponent: With ease, humility, patience, flexibility, spontaneity. These are all qualities of grace.

Grace is as much the *attitude* of an open, patient and lucid mind, as it is the quality of an agile, responsive and coordinated body. In this light, grace arises as the *seamless* interface of an alert, functional mind and an alert, functional body.

Graceful movement arises from the blending of the previous four qualities. The more those qualities are developed and integrated, the more graceful the athlete looks and feels. A graceful athlete is one who is cooperating in a masterful way with his body and with the natural forces of his environment.

How-To: PAGES

Let's identify some ways we can each use our endurance training to craft PAGES movements. Truth is, we have already begun the process - even though we were not aware of PAGES. Already we are:

- Targeting the neural system as a priority in our endurance training.

- More aware of orchestrating and balancing the stress of training with recovery and adaptation. This enables us to consistently gain fitness through the fitness cycle and avoid injury or sickness.

- Sharpening the axe of our perceptive acuity by deliberately and patiently crafting our approach to each training session. This includes both Beginner's and Finalist's Minds.

- Balancing our athletic goal-driven motivation with an appreciation for a more process-oriented (dare I say "artistic"?) pursuit of our craft.

PAGES movements are the tangible results of our patient kaizen-durance craft that enable us to pursue our goals. They are like the thousands of *brush strokes* that a painter crafts upon the canvas of a painting: Each one is part of the final masterpiece.

Here are some ways to explore and refine your PAGES strokes and strides

- Use recovery sessions as your Golden Opportunity.

- With a "Gratitude Attitude", you can find the opportunity to pursue mastery even in the most challenging circumstances. This is an extension of our approach.

- Implement a consistent practice of functional strength training.

• Participate in reputable technique clinics.

Let's consider each of these briefly, beginning with...

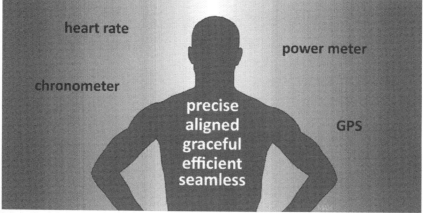

The Golden Opportunity

In Chapter 3, we considered recovery sessions as the Golden Opportunities for honing our Approaching Skills - our skills at sharpening the axe of perceptive acuity and readiness. Our recovery sessions serve also as the perfect "studio" for crafting our very finest Precise, Aligned, Graceful, Efficient and Seamless strokes and strides. Think of each stroke like the stroke of a paint brush on the canvas of a masterpiece painting by Rembrandt. Each one is vital to the overall composition.

Refer again to the guidelines offered in Chapter 3 for conducting your recovery sessions. Once you have paused to sharpen your axe, to summon your Beginner's and/or Finalist's mind, begin your session slow and easy. Again, Rate of Perceived Exertion should be at or below 4-5 on a scale of 1-10.

For each recovery session, you can choose one of the five qualities of PAGES movements and *embody* that one as you train. The BIG question of course is: *"How do I train and evaluate Precise, Aligned, Graceful, Efficient and Seamless movements?"*

The answer to this question is very simple, yet very profound: You must *"listen"*. Turn off that little voice in the penthouse suite of the frontal cortex and *listen to your sense-felt experience*. This is where creativity and intuition can cooperate with logic. Easy enough to say. However, if you have always relied upon "numbers" to guide you through every training session, this may feel like very foreign territory.

Training without your numbers may feel like flying to foreign country after living your whole life in familiar surroundings: You don't speak the language, the food is strange, you are in a different time zone, and you don't know your way around. Be patient, be curious, be aware. Be a Beginner - it's OK!! In the mind of the Beginner, there are infinite possibilities for discovery, in the mind of the Expert, there are very few.

Since you left all those distracting number-producing devices at home - the heart-rate monitor, power meter, GPS, etc - you have freed up lots of bandwidth in your head to focus on what it actually *feels* like to swim, bike or run. You can actually notice the world around you too!

How can you evaluate PAGES? Ultimately you have to *feel* each one. One way to evaluate: As you monitor your Rate of Perceived Exertion, you can strive to relax even more so that your RPE goes down at the same pace, or your pace increases slightly at the same RPE. If you don't yet feel confident to gauge your RPE, use a heart-rate monitor for *occasional* reference.

To summarize, turn off your external measuring devices during your recovery sessions and learn to listen and respond to your own *sense-felt experience.*

dark

rain

hills

wind   alone

late   rough

Challenging Conditions = Opportunity

current   mud

murky

hot

early   waves

cold   MAH

Gratitude Attitude

As you focus on crafting masterful PAGES strokes and strides, you can welcome and embrace things that you perceive as obstacles, and transform them into opportunities. Again, picture the wise old Sensei as he faces his young opponent. He welcomes anger and aggression, responding to them not in kind, but with serenity and ease.

The best opportunity as you bike and run? *Hills!!* For me, hills offer a sort of magnifying glass that I can use to really study my technique. The additional challenge requires *finesse*, not aggression and exertion. Other "adverse" conditions also provide these opportunities: wind, heat, rough open water for swimming, uneven running and biking surfaces... If you find yourself growing annoyed, impatient or resistant, that is a sign that you have an opportunity to challenge and strengthen your approach.

To summarize, embrace inconvenience, challenging terrain and uncomfortable conditions as opportunities to train finer mental and physical skills (collectively your kinetic intelligence). While others may continue wasting energy resisting or fighting adverse conditions, you can empower your relationship to them and pursue mastery.

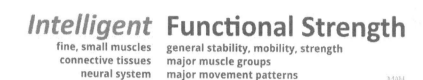

Intelligent **Functional Strength**

fine, small muscles   **general stability, mobility, strength**
connective tissues   **major muscle groups**
neural system   **major movement patterns**   MAH

Functional Strength

I mentioned briefly that stability, mobility and agility are essential tools as you craft PAGES movements. Collectively, these are known as *"functional strength"*. I will go one step further: *"intelligent* functional strength".

Conventionally, we regard strength as well-developed major muscles - the big ones we can see, the ones that do most of the work as we move forward. However, precise, aligned, graceful, efficient and seamless strokes and strides require a finer, more "detailed" kind of strength that ensures stability, mobility and agility.

As active endurance athletes (especially multi-sport athletes), we adequately strengthen our major muscle groups during our actual endurance training. However, intelligent functional strength training is vital for us to avoid injury and improve our PAGES. Traditional Pilates mat work is a great place to start. Specifically we must train both the finer, smaller muscles and connective tissues (ligaments and tendons) of the muscular system, *as well as the neural system*. Pilates mat work encourages the deliberate precision that we need for PAGES.

Challenging the body with stability-limited exercises tasks the neural system with learning exactly which of the finer muscles and connective tissues around the joints to activate for stability. With "stability-limited" exercises, we create conditions which make balance and stability more challenging. As an example: Push-ups with your feet or your hands on a fitness ball.

As we gain neural intelligence, we can then increase the range of motion through which we are maintaining that stability. This becomes functional mobility. An athlete can have great range of motion (flexibility) but may be unable to remain stable throughout that range. Functional mobility is a combination of flexibility and stability.

Agility combines stability and mobility with balance and coordination so we can craft complex and synchronized PAGES movements.

It is well beyond the purview of this introductory book to delve any more into the details of training and developing functional strength. However, I want to emphasize that this form of training targets the *neural* system as much or even more than the muscular. This training process involves giving the neural system a "stability problem" to solve - a problem that we do not normally encounter in our familiar repetitive movement patterns.

It is also essential that you choose problems or tasks that are *appropriate for your current ability*. The emphasis of this *intelligence* training is not on "how many reps" or "how much weight" or "how unstable". It is about facilitating *your* neural system learning how to stabilize in every plane of movement so that your strokes and strides are PAGES, *and so you can remain injury-free*.

In summary, functional strength provides a foundation for your athletic abilities. Functional strength is not merely strength of the major muscles. It is the ability to control your body for safer, stronger movement patterns. This is training that integrates the muscular and neurologic systems together.

Choose to pre-hab so you aren't forced to re-hab.

Technique Programs

It is vital for every athlete to recognize that there is no one single superior swim stroke, pedal stroke or run stride that will work for every athlete: There is no "one-size-fits-all". Each of us embodies a unique combination of abilities and challenges, and each of us must patiently navigate our individual way on the path of mastery. Therefore, each of us will develop our own unique technique.

However, there are essential fundamental biomechanical elements that *every* swimmer, biker and runner will embody. (One example is alignment.) Each of us then adapts these fundamental elements to our unique "instrument". These fundamentals elements are based on the physics of each sport - on the universal laws (arising as forces) that are "at play" in each moment. The primary force that informs our technique for every form of movement? Gravity, of course. Therefore, *all* of us must explore and build upon common technique fundamentals as we craft PAGES strokes and strides.

The most valuable assets we can acquire from a technique clinic are:

- Identify the fundamental biomechanical elements specific to the sport and the universal laws that govern those elements

- Acquire effective navigational skills and tools that empower us to explore and experience the fundamental biomechanical elements through sense-felt experience

- Feedback (via insightful observation from a coach) on how we are perceiving and responding to these elements; not only to correct our movements, but also to improve our perceptive acuity so that we can self-correct

- Acquire effective navigational tools so that we can evaluate PAGES through (internal) sense-felt experience and through (external) metrics

These navigational skills and tools empower us to successfully pursue that perfect run stride, that perfect pedal stroke, that perfect swim stroke for *this present moment* - the one that feels effortless and graceful in this environment, on this terrain. We acquire these navigational aides through:

- A sharper axe (improved perceptive acuity)

- Clear comprehension (both in mind and body) of the laws of physics that are at play as we swim/bike/run etc

- Drills

- Sensation-based focal points

- Visualization techniques

- Shifts in our approach

...And remember: This is a pursuit of mastery. There is no permanent finish line. Don't be discouraged by this! Instead, embrace the incredible opportunity: While our aerobic capacity will diminish, we can refine our *craft* indefinitely.

Kinetic Intelligence Revisited

To summarize, kinetic intelligence is the awareness and the skill to occupy and animate our bodies with precision, grace and ease. It includes:

- The ability to clearly perceive how we are moving right now

- The skill to "problem-solve" in the moment so that we can adapt and refine our movements

- The ability to clearly imprint and reliably recall these new, wiser movements

Our popular notion of intelligence "locates" it in our brains. But what is intelligence really? I offer that it is our ability to perceive and observe events and to *draw relationships* between those events. Our brain is a complex matrix of cells that are "wired" together via neurons. The cells are the "events" and the neural network comprises the relationships between these.

Kinetic intelligence is essentially the same thing. However, the complex matrix now includes not just the cells of the brain, but *the cells of the body as well*. This form of intelligence engages the *entire neural system* as it connects brain and body. Hence, the emphasis on athletically training our neural system.

PAGES strokes and strides arise from kinetic intelligence. Like other aspects of intelligence, through consistent lifelong study and acquisition, it becomes a form of *wisdom* we cultivate with age. Like other forms of intelligence and knowledge, effective acquisition requires good habits and practices. And… I'll say it once again, this begins with the sharp axe of perceptive acuity and a diligent, patient and mindful approach. (A dose of playful, curious creativity also enhances that acquisition significantly.)

Chapter Summary

Kinetic intelligence becomes the wisdom of the master athlete. This is what we stand to gain as we age beyond prime aerobic capacity. Patience, humility and perseverance are precious virtues in this lifelong acquisition.

The notion that mastery requires ten thousand repetitions is not absolute. With a patient and mindful approach and a very sharp axe of perceptive acuity, our practice is ever closer to perfection, from the very first repetition.

Our neural system responds and improves the most to training. Neural plasticity is the measure of our potential for improving. We deliberately use our *approach* as a means of optimizing neural plasticity. With a high degree of neural plasticity, we no longer require ten thousand repetitions. To put it in contemporary terms, with neural plasticity we can "hack" kinetic intelligence.

We have begun to explore the possibility of *effortless power*. To "play" with effortless power, we must embrace the "Paradox of Control": We cannot control the circumstances that are arising in each moment. However, we can *choose* to seek the opportunity that is arising in these circumstances. We can choose to embrace and to orchestrate the forces that are "at play" rather than resisting them.

As master athletes, we embrace the forces that are arising and - with our wisdom - use them to patiently advance.

PAGES movements are the craft we practice with our kinetic intelligence. The "build sequence" is:

- Aligned

- Precise

- Seamless

- Efficient

- Graceful

Each one supports and facilitates the next.

To excel as master athletes we pursue PAGES in our strokes and strides. To do this, we:

- Prioritize neural training in our sessions

- Orchestrate and balance stress with recovery and adaptation

- Invest each day in sharpening the axe of our perceptive acuity as we deliberately and patiently craft our approach to each training session. This includes both Beginner's and Finalist's Minds.

- Balance our athletic goal-driven motivation with an appreciation for a process-oriented pursuit of our craft.

Ways to explore and refine PAGES:

- Use recovery sessions as your Golden Opportunity

- With a "Gratitude Attitude", you can find the opportunity to pursue mastery even in the most challenging circumstances. This is an extension of our approach

- Implement a consistent practice of functional strength training

- Participate in reputable technique clinics

Every form of intelligence is alive within us as an interactive matrix of events. Our neural system functions as that matrix. Kinetic intelligence engages the entire neural system, networking both brain and body.

What's Next?

In our explorations of effortless power and PAGES movements, I have mentioned a *force* that is constantly available to each of us. Honoring the Paradox of Control, we accept that we cannot control or conquer this force. However, we can channel this force and use it to move us forward, so that we are able to conserve our energy and minimize the need to generate our own force.

This force also provides us with essential orientation for Alignment - the first element of the PAGES strokes and strides of the master athlete. Without this force, we would be floating in a sea of confusion and disorientation. Literally.

CHAPTER SIX

GRAVITY: SOURCE OF EFFORTLESS POWER

Precession

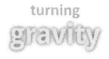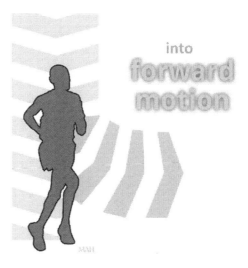

Effortless Power: Myth or Method?

The paradoxical term *"effortless power"* was coined decades ago by one of the greatest contemporary martial arts masters, Peter Ralston. (I had the great fortune to study with Peter for a few months when he was "on sabbatical" in Hawaii.) Peter is the only non-Asian to win the full-contact Martial Arts World Championship that used to be held annually in China. People died in this tournament over the years.

In his peak competitive era, Peter had the reputation of fighting like a *drunken sailor*. He would enter the ring and simply stand in front of his opponent - completely relaxed and empty, no fighting pose. Yet, underneath that emptiness and relaxation lay extraordinary perceptive acuity and agility. Peter claims that in this state, he can often perceive exactly what his opponent is about to do... *before his opponent knows!* Truly, if we approach with a sharp axe, there are no limits to our perceptive acuity. Given this skill, Peter can easily embrace and redirect his opponent's force back at him.

Like Peter Ralston and the wise old masters portrayed in Karate Kid and King Fu, as master athletes we too can tap into forces "at play" as we train and race. We too can gracefully redirect and orchestrate those forces to patiently and efficiently advance towards our goals. And similar to the martial arts arena, the primary force we can partner with also appears initially as an *opponent*.

As master athletes, the force we align with is...

Gravity

Many athletes regard gravity as an opponent, as a force to deny, to fight against. These athletes approach their events as brash and brawny gladiators, ready to conquer gravity, and every other athlete. The simple truth is, none of us will ever conquer gravity. (Nor will we conquer every other athlete.)

Relentlessly, gravity anchors our bodies to Earth's surface - regardless of age, gender, socioeconomic status, ethnicity... It is a sober equalizer. Gravity acts upon (and within) every cell, every molecule, every atom, every sub-atomic particle of our being from the time we are conceived in the womb until the time we leave the body.

Gravity is the great bane of runners - a force that results in impact, the cause of virtually every running injury. In the martial arts arena, an opponent's force can also result in impact. However, the Sensei is able to skillfully embrace and gracefully redirect his opponent's force - easily avoiding impact. With PAGES running strides, we too can redirect and transform the force of gravity from impact into effortless forward momentum.

Without gravity, it is not possible for us to run, to walk, or to intentionally move in any direction.

The very heart and soul of our craft as kaizen-durance athletes is our *alliance with gravity*. In simplest terms, through this alliance, we transform the vertical and inward pull of gravity by 90 degrees into horizontal and forward motion. (Inward meaning towards Earth's center.) Our greatest opponent becomes our greatest ally - a rich and infinite resource - for going faster and further.

Gravity is My Sensei

This introduction to gravity as our source of effortless power, as our essential guide for PAGES may sound extreme at first. However, the simple and profound truth is, for each and every one of us - athletic or not - our relationship with gravity is the most enduring and constant relationship of our lives. (Again, from the time we are conceived, until we leave the body.) We have a lifelong opportunity to *listen* to and align with gravity, to use this force as our primary source of momentum and our most trusted guide. There is no more powerful source of orientation in our lives.

Gravity *is* my Sensei.

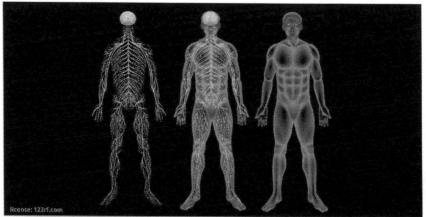

license: 123rf.com

Your Secret Weapon: Proprioception

Throughout this book, we are looking to the wise old Sensei for insight and inspiration as we navigate our kaizen-durance path of mastery. We recognize that his effortless power begins with his perceptive acuity, as well as his patience and his appreciation for harmony and balance.

As master athletes, the source of our effortless power is gravity. To craft a powerful alliance with gravity, we must first be able to *perceive* it. This is a challenge since we cannot see it, hear it, touch it, smell it, or taste it. However, we do *feel* it. We feel the pull of gravity *within* our bodies.

Our ability to *feel* gravity is the most valuable perceptive acuity we can cultivate as master athletes - guiding us every moment in our quest to craft PAGES strokes and strides. This is the perceptive capacity that leads us to effortless power. Our ability to feel gravity and use it for orientation arises from our *proprioception*.

Have you ever paused to really *feel* gravity? Even if you have never invested your full attention to perceiving gravity, your moment-to-moment survival depends on it: After all, your alliance with gravity began in earnest when you first learned to stand up, and then to walk. We call our alliance with gravity "*balance*". Without balance, unable to stand or walk, where would you be?

While we can't see gravity, our vision does provide us with cues that we use for balance. To find out how much you rely on your vision: Balance on one foot, and then close your eyes. A bit more challenging? Without your eyesight, you are now relying solely on two other ways of balancing. These are your vestibular and proprioceptive, both *inner feelings*. Your vestibular organs are located in your inner ears. In simplest terms, they act like a bubble leveling device - similar to the kind a builder uses to check for the horizontal and vertical levels of a structure.

We also rely on our *proprioceptive system* for our alliance with gravity. Proprioceptors are located in every joint and muscle. There are several thousand of these receptors throughout our bodies. They are constantly sending information to our central nervous system about:

- Degree of flexion/extension (joints)

- Degree of tension - that is, contraction/extension (muscles)

- Position and spacial location relative to other proprioceptors

- Direction and speed of motion

- Position and spacial location relative to *the pull of gravity*

These receptors are constantly sending *thousands of signals per second* to the central nervous system. In fact, Nobel laureate Robert Sperry (neuropsychologist and neurobiologist) claimed that these proprioceptive signals comprise *ninety percent* of the neural activity between your body and your brain! (That leaves just ten percent for texting and driving.) Here is a tremendous opportunity for sharpening the axe of our perceptive acuity. And this is the axe that will empower us most as master endurance athletes.

In summary, since we depend upon our proprioception to feel gravity. Improving this perceptive ability is the key to strengthening our alliance with gravity.

How-To: Sharpening The Proprioceptive Axe

It may seem bewildering that proprioceptive awareness doesn't really show up on your radar screen of everyday consciousness. That is, until you walk out the front door on a winter morning and lose your balance on a patch of ice. At this instant, you are no longer thinking about your "To-Do" list, or what music you will listen to on the way to work. At this moment, you are very, very aware of your proprioception as you strive to regain balance.

You don't have to create a sudden crisis of imbalance - like slipping on ice - to invest your full attention on proprioception. Here are some of the ways I invest my awareness and attention to improve proprioception:

- Stability limited exercises

- "Blind Walking"

- Open water swimming, mixed terrain biking and running

- "Falling into speed"

All of these will challenge your proprioceptive balance. Before we briefly explore each of these, let's cover a few "environmental factors" that enhance proprioception.

Relax and Trust Gravity

You see best when your eyes are open, yes? That's obvious. Not so obvious: Proprioception functions best when there is minimal tension in the muscles as well as the connective tissues around the joints. Tension impedes proprioceptive neural function, just as eyelids or dirty glasses impede vision. Our nerves are not able to clearly conduct the electrical signals that comprise proprioception through tense muscles and connective tissues. Tension also requires more energy - diminishing efficiency and therefore endurance and speed.

Relaxation and proprioception enhance one another:

- When we are relaxed, we optimize proprioceptive acuity.

- With that acuity, we align better with gravity - that is, both our static and dynamic balance improve.

- Through this improved alliance with gravity: Our bones support our weight… and we can relax even more.

- With that increased relaxation, the cycle continues as our proprioceptive acuity increases even more.

Let's look at this on a deeper, subtler level: When we stand on one leg, our typical response is to contract the muscles of the supporting leg. That contraction is tension that impedes proprioception. However, with patient *neural* training, we can learn how to stand *through* rather than *on* the supporting leg. What's the difference? When we stand *through* the hip, upper leg, knee, lower leg, ankle and foot, we:

- Align well with gravity so that our bones can support most of the weight

- Avoid *contracting* the major muscles and instead, we allow them to *compress*

There is a subtle, yet quite profound difference between contracting and compressing the muscles. With patient neural training, we can discern the difference, and learn to minimize muscular contraction. This is a profound skill for endurance efficiency - one largely disregarded in conventional training methods.

Compression is passive - requiring no energy. Contraction is active - requiring energy. If we can minimize the contractile response of every running stride over the course of a marathon, we:

- Conserve lots of energy

- Align better with gravity through enhanced proprioception

- Decrease impact due to improved alignment and better absorption through relaxed, compressing muscles

- Run with optimal PAGES strides

Benefits of Proprioceptive Acuity

As you gain proprioceptive acuity, you will

- Exert less energy

- Go further and/or faster

- Significantly reduce your risk of injury (especially the impact of running)

- Recover faster

- Improve your PAGES strokes and strides

Proprioceptive awareness has kept me virtually injury free over four decades of running. In the past few years (I'm in my late-50's), I have wrapped up my season each year in late-November to early-December with consecutive weekly distance running events:

- 2013: Single/Double/Triple marathons: (Week 1: Philadelphia Marathon, Week 2: JFK 50-Mile (plus 2.4 miles), Week 3: NCR Trail Marathon (same course 3 days in a row)

- 2014 & 2015: JFK 50-Mile, NCR Trail Marathon, 100-Mile Run (2014: Cajun Coyote 100, 2015: Hitchcock 100)

- 2018: JFK 50-Mile and Philadelphia Marathon on consecutive days, NCR Trail Marathon 6 days later

Below I offer a brief discussion of each of the ways we can improve proprioceptive awareness.

Stability-Limited Exercises

Already mentioned in the last chapter, there are many simple exercises we can do to vastly improve joint stability - especially *lateral* joint stability in the hips and feet. Lateral stability begins with proprioception. Choose the most minimal foot wear that is appropriate for you to target foot stability.

Single Leg Squats:

- Begin in a Standing Athletic Position, flexed at hips and knees, with flat back, aligned spine, feet parallel at hip width

- Maintain this stance as you shift all your weight to one foot (right foot)

- Lift unweighted (left) foot slightly behind you and position opposite (right arm) on lower back

- You now look like a speed skater, with arms and legs vertically aligned

- Visually spot on the floor a meter or two ahead

- Slowly lower by your body by flexing more at hip, knee and ankle of supporting foot, *not* by tipping your torso forward

- Keep knee vertically aligned over foot, without allowing your knee to extend out past your toes

- Slowly raise back up to a slightly flexed (not straight) knee

- Repeat 6-10 times and then return to Standing Athletic Position and switch to other leg

- Emphasize alignment and precision, keeping the exercise slow

Watch me demonstrate this exercise in this brief video: https://www.dropbox.com/s/acizgfae4jna4en/SLS.MOV?dl=0

Leg Swings:

- Begin in same Standing Athletic Position, and again shift to Speed Skater Stance, balancing on one leg (left), this time with back arm (left) and hand positioned in swing position, not resting on low back

- Begin to swing (right) leg and opposite (left) arm front to back as you counterbalance that swing with your torso and (right) arm swinging forward, everything pivoting on hip of supporting leg

- Keep knee of supporting leg bent

- Minimize tension in supporting foot

- Relax into swing, focusing on the counterbalance of arms, legs and torso, and vertical alignment of arms and legs

- Do 6-20 swings and then return to Standing Athletic Position and switch to other leg

- The more relaxed your joints and muscles, the easier this will be

- As you relax, you will be able to increase the range of motion of the swing

Watch me demonstrate this exercise in this brief video: https://www.dropbox.com/s/6lyfmnd1n3vefm4/LegSwing.MOV?dl=0

Balance Disc:

Spend a few minutes 2 or 3 times a week on a balance disc or wobble board. Challenge your balance by:

- Squatting up and down slowly with both feet wide apart on disc
- Without squatting, fan arms up and down like jumping jacks
- Fan arms front to back at shoulder height
- Single leg squats, with standing foot at center of disc
- Same fanning arm movements balancing on single leg

Watch me demonstrate this exercise in this brief video: https://www.dropbox.com/s/dtplbfx2qi1w7sw/Disc.MOV?dl=0

"Blind Walking"

Blind Walking is very simple, yet very profound. It is a moving meditation. Close your eyes and walk very, very slowly. This exercise is an excellent way to neurally train muscular compression instead muscular contraction as you slowly weight each hip/leg/foot.

- Find a quiet place with a level floor
- Close your eyes and stand for at least one minute, knees relaxed and slightly flexed, feet parallel and shoulder width
- Lengthen your low back/spine by slightly tipping your pelvis
- Feel as if there is a thin cable attached to the crown of your head that is gently pulling you to the ceiling
- Bring your awareness to your breathing
- Feel the energy rise through your body on the inhale
- Feel the energy fall through your body on the exhale
- Relax your feet: Feel as if the soles of your feet are like soft butter melting into a warm pan
- When you feel calm and aware of your body, slowly shift all your

weight to one hip/leg/foot, keeping it relaxed

- Now slowly shift your weight to the other hip/leg/foot

- Repeat this slow and simple weight shift

- To focus on compressing instead of contracting the muscles of your hip/leg/foot (as discussed above), shift your awareness to your empty hip/leg/foot before you begin to "pour" your weight into itFeel the relaxation in this empty side and then slowly pour your weight through your hip, leg, ankle and foot

- Feel the weight drain through the sole of your foot into the earth

- When you are ready to do this walking, slowly peel the unweighted foot off the floor (peeling off heel to toe)

- Advance the foot forward as you inhale and set it down gently and slowly without weighting it until it is completely on the floor

- Now, slowly pour your weight into it as you exhale

- Repeat the same pattern for a slow walk

- As you walk, articulate the flexion/extension of your knees to keep your pelvis level side-to-side

- Use the knee articulation to also keep your height constant: No bobbing up and down as you walk

- If you are walking in a small space, you may need to pause and turn around every few steps

- Keep your movements slow and seamless

You may notice the tendency to rush the foot forward once you have lifted it off the ground. This is the most challenging phase of the walk, as you balance *through* one hip, leg, ankle and foot. I choose the word "through" instead of "on". When we relax, we allow the weight to pour through the bones and compressed muscles, instead of locking it in tense muscles.

For a detailed video demonstration, you can purchase my "Tai Chi for Athletes" DVD.

Mixed Terrain

A majority of endurance events - particularly triathlons - are limited to paved roads for cycling and running. And for most of us, that's also where we train. However, running exclusively on pavement significantly increases the risk of injuries and does not challenge proprioception or lateral joint stability as much as mixed terrain.

While there are less gains to be had with mixed terrain cycling for conventional multisport athletes who compete on paved surfaces (and an increase in risk of injury), it does challenge proprioception and bike handling skills. Improving handling skills may make the difference between successfully negotiating an obstacle or crashing during a race or training ride on the road.

With swimming, it's the opposite. We train in a pool - with a flat surface - but we compete in open water - with a constantly varying surface. Let's start with swimming.

Open Water Swimming:

- If you are preparing for an event with an open-water swim, there is no substitute: practice swimming in open water. The calm flat surface of a pool does little to prepare us for the chop, wind, swells and currents of open water. These all affect vestibular balance.

- The pool provides visual cues for balance and orientation that are absent out in the ocean or lake. Lack of visual cues and vestibular confusion challenge us to rely more on proprioceptive balance.

- Varying surface conditions require constant flexibility and adaptation in stroke technique, stroke length and cadence.

Mixed Terrain Running:

- Constantly varying terrain and pitch challenge proprioceptive balance and response time with every stride and foot contact

- Requires constant variation and flexibility in stride technique, stride length and cadence

- Variety diminishes the risk of overuse injuries.

- Constant variation requires full attention - no "auto-pilot" allowed!

Mixed Terrain Cycling:

- The most popular form is mountain biking; however, over technical terrain, without adequate handling skills, this can result in injuries

- Choose terrain suitable to your skill level and equipment

- Hard-packed unpaved roads may be suitable for a road bike, with lower tire pressure

- Even hilly paved roads serve well

- When riding over challenging sections, or climbing hills, shift your weight smoothly from pedal-to-pedal, and keep your arms and upper body relaxed

"Fall Into Speed"

As we convert the vertical pull of gravity into horizontal motion, we can "fall into speed". As an example, while running, as we lean forward, we begin to *fall* forward. We craft our strides so that our feet land very slightly behind the tipping point of that fall. With this dynamic balance, we are as close to perpetual motion as we can get. As we lean forward (from the ankles, not the waist), we "fall into speed". The more we lean the faster we can go. However the "edge" of that balance begins to get sharper and more difficult to maintain.

We can also fall into speed as we swim and bike. To explore these, refer to "The Swimmer's Dilemma" and "The Cyclist's Dilemma" on the Kaizen-durance website.

Falling into speed begins with our approach. We patiently begin each training session by relaxing deeply and tapping into our proprioception. At the start, we strive to keep our Perceived Rate of Exertion as low as possible: We want to first optimize our alliance with gravity, before we begin to add any additional force of our own. This is true for swimming and cycling, as well as running.

Falling into speed becomes part of our patient approach.

Gravity-Based Propulsion

In the previous chapter, I suggested technique clinics as a way to explore and refine our PAGES movements. In light of what we have considered in this chapter, seek out technique clinics that focus on *gravity-based propulsion*. Our PAGES movements are based first on optimizing our alliance with gravity:

- We begin with Alignment. The primary reference or guidance we use for alignment is our perception of gravity.

- The quality of Precision in our movements is also determined by our dynamic relationship (balance) with gravity.

- Efficiency arises from less effort and exertion, as we learn to "fall" forward.

- Seamless movements maintain the delicate dynamic balance of falling forward.

- Grace is the synergy of all of these qualities, as well as an attitude of gentleness, patience and ease - even in the most challenging moments

In my many years of teaching swimming, cycling and occasionally running technique, alliance with gravity is always the primary orientation.

Chapter Summary

The expression "effortless power" is a paradox: How can we generate power with no effort? It becomes less paradoxical when we honor the Paradox of Control: Instead of struggling to control the forces that are at play, we embrace them and redirect them to patiently and efficiently advance towards our goals.

The force that is most at play as we train and race is gravity. It acts upon and within us at the most macro and micro levels of existence during every moment of our lives.

We can choose to regard gravity as an opponent, and struggle (in vain) to conquer it. Or, we can commit to a lifelong alliance with gravity that grows stronger with age and experience.

The very heart and soul of our craft as Kaizen-durance athletes is our *alliance with gravity*. In simplest terms, through this alliance, we transform the vertical and inward pull of gravity by 90 degrees into horizontal and forward motion. Our greatest opponent becomes our greatest ally - a rich and infinite resource - for going faster and further.

To craft a powerful alliance with gravity, we must first be able to *perceive* it. Yet, we cannot see it, hear it, touch it, smell it, or taste it. However, we do *feel* the pull of gravity *within us*. Our ability to *feel* gravity is the most valuable perceptive acuity we can cultivate as master athletes. Our ability to feel gravity is called *proprioception*.

73

Throughout our lives, many of us have never paused to *feel* gravity. However, since infancy, we have been feeling gravity *"in the back of our minds"* to maintain balance. We use three senses for balance:

- Vision

- Vestibular

- Proprioception

Proprioceptors are constantly informing our central nervous system about:

- Degree of flexion/extension (joints)

- Degree of tension - that is, contraction/extension (muscles)

- Position and spacial location relative to other proprioceptors

- Direction and speed of motion

- Position and spacial location relative to the pull of gravity

These receptors send *thousands of signals per second* to the central nervous system, and comprise perhaps *ninety percent* of the neural activity between your body and your brain! Training proprioceptive awareness is a tremendous opportunity for sharpening the axe of our perceptive acuity. And this is the axe that will empower us most as master endurance athletes.

To train proprioceptivity, include these activities in your training:

- Stability limited exercises

- "Blind Walking"

- Open water swimming, mixed terrain biking and running

- "Falling into speed"

We usually respond to weight and impact with muscular tension. This tension impedes proprioception just at the critical moment of footfall as we run. And tension requires more energy.

With patient *neural* training, we can learn how to stand *through* rather than *on* the supporting leg. That is respond by allowing the major muscles to *compress* rather than contract. Compression is passive - requiring no energy. Contraction is active - requiring energy. This is a profound skill for endurance efficiency - one largely disregarded in conventional training methods.

As you gain proprioceptive acuity, you will

- Conserve energy

- Go further and/or faster

- Reduce risk of injury (especially the impact of running)

- Recover faster

- Improve PAGES strokes and strides

When we dynamically align with gravity, we "fall into speed" by converting the vertical pull of gravity into horizontal motion. At the beginning of each training session, with a patient approach, we start by tuning into our perception of gravity and optimizing our alliance with gravity. Keeping the PRE low, we relax and fall into speed.

Efficiency-focused technique clinics are built upon *gravity-based propulsion*. Likewise, PAGES movements are based first on optimizing our alliance with gravity:

- We begin with Alignment. The primary reference or orientation we use for alignment is our perception of gravity.

- The quality of Precision in our movements is also determined by our dynamic relationship (balance) with gravity.

- Efficiency arises from less effort and exertion, as we learn to "fall" forward.

- Seamless movements maintain the delicate dynamic balance of falling forward.

- Grace is the synergy of all of these qualities, as well as an attitude of gentleness, patience and ease - even in the most challenging moments.

What's Next?

All of the elements of kaizen-durance that we have explored so far require that we fully occupy and engage in this present moment, here and now. The most essential training that enables us to do this is *mindfulness training*. As action-oriented beings, we endurance athletes are not so fond of something that appears to be so passive and so tedious.

In fact, or training is often a way to escape the problems that we face in the "here-and-now" of our lives. However, mindfulness training can significantly enhance our athletic performance. Is can also empower us to embrace and respond to the challenges of our daily lives, instead of resisting and fighting them.

In the next chapter, we explore the riches of mindfulness training. Mindfulness ensures that we maximize return on our aerobic investment.

CHAPTER SEVEN:
MINDFULNESS: ULTIMATE BASE TRAINING

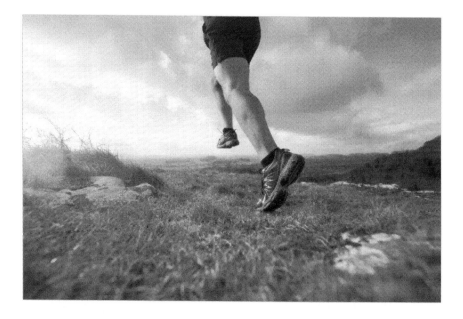

No, It Doesn't Make Sense

Throughout this book, we have looked at some things that seem contradictory, even absurd:

- A wise old Sensei who wastes his time trying to catch flies with chopsticks

- A world champion martial arts master who enters the ring like a drunken sailor

- Waxing cars and painting fences to learn karate

- Expressions like "effortless power", "paradox of control", and "falling into speed"

- Approaching athletic training more like a musician preparing to play a symphony than a gladiator with his eyes on the prize

And yet, in the Pursuit of Mastery, each of these oddities serves a purpose and reveals some insight. In this chapter, we will explore something that may initially appear the most contradictory and absurd of all.

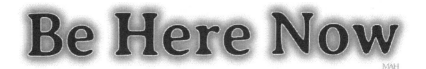

Be Here Now

What does it really mean to "sharpen the axe" of perceptive acuity? How do we actually *do* this? Can we identify a specific activity - an effective, reliable technique if you will - that enables us to maximize perceptive acuity, to be hyper-aware?

Let's return to *"kaizen"* - continuous life improvement: To pursue mastery in any and every area of life, we relentlessly (yet patiently) challenge and train our perceptive acuity. That's it. (The brilliance of mastery arises from this perceptive acuity.) And it's important to remember that the opportunity to pursue mastery exists in *every moment and circumstance of our lives* - the good ones and the bad ones just the same.

A master does not really *know more* than someone else. Instead, a master more accurately perceives what is unfolding here and now, and can therefore respond brilliantly.

At the most stripped-down, bare-bones level, we can express this in three one syllable words: BE HERE NOW. Generously invest our awareness and attention in *this present moment.* Fully engage in *this present moment.* Unconditionally. When we "Be Here Now", mastery simply arises.

To sharpen the axe, we must train our awareness and attention to be here in this present moment - regardless of what is occurring. This is called *mindfulness training.* This is the hard-core essence of mastery and kaizen - as mundane as it appears.

Simple Exercise

Here is perhaps the most effective mindfulness training technique in the world. It's been around for more than a thousand years. Nothing could be simpler than this:

- Find a quiet place, with no visual or auditory distractions.

- Set a timer for 8 minutes. (Traditionally, it's for a minimum 20 minutes, but let's go easy here.)

- Sit comfortably - on a chair, or on the floor.

- Your spine is aligned, lengthened.

- Keep your pelvic core and low back engaged to maintain your long aligned spine.

- Tuck your chin, lengthen the back of your neck.

- Rest your hands in your lap or on your knees.

- Open or close your eyes.

- Start the timer.

- Breathe slowly through your nose.

- Lightly rest the tip of your tongue along the gum line of your top front teeth.

- Keep your attention and awareness on your breath - each inhale, each exhale - for 8 minutes.

- When you realize that your attention has drifted away, gently return it to your breath.

That's it. That's the supreme ancient practice of training mindfulness known as *"sitting meditation"*: Stay present with your breathing and *observe* what your mind does. How long before your attention wanders from your breath to:

- The past?
- The future?
- A fear?
- A desire?
- A judgment?
- An obligation or commitment, or…

It is the nature of the untrained mind (traditionally called *"monkey mind"*) to wander from one thing to the next. Yet, when it wanders, we lose our perceptive acuity about what is unfolding here and now. Or we cloud and distort those perceptions with fears, desires, judgments, etc.

The training in this practice is simple: When you realize your attention has drifted to something else, gently return to your breathing. You are not really training the monkey mind that wanders. You are training the awareness that is "outside" this monkey mind.

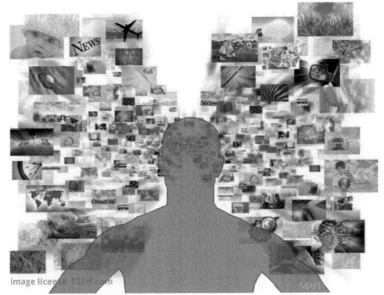

Awareness and Attention

Throughout this book I often pair the words "*awareness*" and "*attention*". Why not simply use one word or the other? Awareness and attention are not the same, and both are essential for perceptive acuity.

Attention is our perception of what we are focusing on right now. This can be a sense-felt experience, a thought, an emotion, or some combination of these. The undisciplined monkey mind can shift our attention in an instant, jumping from one thing to another.

Awareness is our consciousness *outside* of this attention. With this awareness, we are able to monitor the activity and focus or our attention. As we strengthen awareness, we are able to more effectively articulate and direct our attention - like a tool.

Through mindfulness training, we first awaken to this awareness that is outside of the incessant activity of our immediate attention. We become familiar with the subtle, silent, calm and still "landscape" of this awareness. As we begin to inhabit and find grounding in this landscape, we gain the perceptive strength to use our attention like a tool. No longer does it wander hither and yon so often.

Awakening to our awareness and successfully interfacing it with our attention is quite rigorous, even though it appears as if we are *not doing or accomplishing anything!* It is seen as a practice of *non-doing* - of simply *being*. That is, with both awareness and attention, we are *being here now*.

The Ultimate Approach

And so, here we are considering another contradiction: How can such a passive practice of *doing nothing* help us in the pursuit of mastery... in anything? As contradictory as it seems, the value for us as master athletes is already apparent. That rigorous practice of non-doing is the ultimate way to sharpen the axe of perceptive acuity:

- Pause to "locate and inhabit" your awareness.

- From your awareness, find the "handle" of your attention so that you can control it as a tool.

- With this "awareness-attention-interface" complete, your axe is sharp and ready.

Mindfulness training enables us to reliably and consistently orchestrate our Approach. Mindfulness ensures that we maximize the return on our aerobic investment.

In this practice of "doing nothing but sitting and breathing", we are awakening a clear, empty and still awareness outside of our monkey mind. It is precisely this *clear empty mind state* of awareness that gives Peter Ralston the hyper-awareness in the fighting ring to perceive what his opponent is going to do *before his opponent knows!* And yes, Peter has invested many hours in the *non-doing* of sitting meditation.

We too can benefit from this clear empty mind state of awareness as master athletes. With such hyper awareness, we are able to precisely adjust each stoke and stride for maximum PAGES. We are able to precisely adjust our pace and metabolic intensity even at the early stages of a very long race so that we can finish strong instead of DNF.

It is natural for us to feel a strong aversion to sitting meditation. (Picture a monkey in a small cage.) After all, what's the goal? How do we measure progress? How can we make time to simply sit and *do nothing* when we can barely juggle the activities of each day and get in enough endurance training? The whole notion of sitting around and doing nothing is in opposition to how we live. If our intention is to fully engage, then sitting and doing nothing but observing our breathing seems lazy and unproductive. We are athletes!! There are laps to swim, hills to bike, miles to run.

A Little Personal History

I confess here and now: I have practiced precious little sitting meditation in my life. And yet, in the past 4 decades, a daily practice of *mindful movement* has sharpened my axe of perceptive acuity significantly: I am able to consistently inhabit the calm, still and empty "landscape" of awareness outside the monkey mind and to patiently and gently direct my attention.

My lifelong study and practice of mindful movement started at age 19, with my collegiate study of modern dance, my job at UPS, recreational running, and the practice of T'ai Chi. (Yes, I treated my job as a package handler in a large UPS truck terminal as an opportunity to study movement just as earnestly as my collegiate pursuit of Modern Dance.) While I danced (and worked for UPS) for just 10 years, I continue T'ai Chi and mindful running to this day.

Over twenty years later, after living in Kona Hawaii for 8 years, I finally witnessed Ironman in 1998, as a volunteer at an aid station on the run course. There and then, I made the resolution that I was going to cross that Hawaii Ironman finish line one year later. Yet, *I had never done a triathlon!* I felt confident that my two decades of mindful movement practice would compensate for my complete lack of experience with triathlon. This would be my one-year experiment.

(Note: I must add that, as a Big Island resident, I was entitled to compete for one of the thirty local Hawaii Ironman slots. All I had to do was qualify for that slot at the Keauhou Half-Iron in May 1999 in a field of sixty locals - far better odds than non-islanders vying for a Kona slot.)

I succeeded in finishing Hawaii Ironman one year later, after some hard-learned lessons that almost cost me my life. In the nearly two decades since then, I have devoted much of my time and energy to developing and practicing the craft of kaizen-durance, and sharing that craft and my insights with others:

- Embedding the practice of mindfulness and the pursuit of mastery in endurance training and racing.

- Balancing that mindful training and racing with the practice of mindfulness and pursuit of mastery in every area of life - in short...

- Balancing the glorious athlete with the ordinary, healthy human being.

-    With this new insight on mindfulness as the core of kaizen-durance - the ultimate base training - let's look again at how we can sharpen that axe of perceptive acuity:

- During our daily endurance training

- Through some more traditional simple practices

- During our day-to-day activities outside of training

Formal or Informal: Black Tie or Barefoot?

Every moment of our lives we have the opportunity to hone mindfulness skills so that we can experience kaizen lifelong improvement in our relationships, occupations, goals and accomplishments, even in the most ordinary and mundane daily tasks. We sharpen that axe through both formal and informal practice.

In formal practice, simply *being here now* is our primary intention and objective - with no ulterior motive or purpose. For instance, sitting meditation has no apparent practical value, no externally measurable benefit. We are just sitting and - on the surface - "*doing nothing*". As we considered earlier, this can be a "tough sell" in our hyperactive lives. However, traditional formal practice *is the most rigorous and effective way* to strengthen our awareness and interface that awareness with our attention so we can sharpen perceptive acuity.

On the other hand, with informal practice, we approach any activity as an opportunity to invest our full awareness and attention to what is arising. There is no formal context, no deliberate or explicit mindfulness preparation as we engage in the activities of the day. Through informal practice, we are embracing each moment, as it arises - ordinary or extraordinary - as the *only opportunity we have right now* to engage with and to train mindfulness.

This moment here and now is the *only* moment we have. We cannot live in the past or in the future.

To clarify formal and informal practice let's consider some examples of each.

Formal Practice

Here are some opportunities for traditional formal practice:

- Sitting meditation

- Yoga and Body Scan

- Simple T'ai Chi

Sitting meditation: We have already considered the starkly simple practice of sitting meditation: Sit with a straight spine, and observe your breath. When you realize your mind has wandered, gently return your awareness to your breath. This is the most direct way to sharpen your axe. You are awakening to an observer *outside* of your attention-mind that can learn how that attention-mind works and how to use it more effectively as a tool.

Can you devote even 5 minutes a day - in the quiet of the early morning, or just before your training, or in the quiet of the evening - to this simple practice? Try it for 30 days. Expect and accept that your attention-mind will stray often from the present moment and from the breath. This is the nature of the mind. "Success" is not measured in controlling our thoughts or preventing our attention from wandering. Rather, we seek to develop a calm and quiet awareness that can observe the attention-mind and its behavior.

Many years ago, I read a short interview with Paula Newby-Fraser in Tricycle, a magazine about mindfulness. At that time, Paula was at the height of her career as a professional triathlete, a multiple Hawaii Ironman

World Champion. In that interview, Paula stated that sitting in meditation was, for her, far more challenging than training for and competing in Hawaii Ironman.

Developing the *strong still, deep and quiet awareness* that can observe the attention-mind and learn to use it as a tool is a lifelong pursuit. It is also the secret of brilliance (something we will explore in Kaizen-durance Book 5: "Brilliance and Flow State".

Yoga and body scan: Our untrained minds are like monkeys that are suddenly set free after being caged. They run and dart about in all directions, with no apparent control or focus: Our minds will slip into the past, project into the future, and produce incessant commentary about anything and everything. Our bodies however, only know and exist in the *present moment*. Our bodies are experts at Being Here Now.

The word "*yoga*" means "*yoke*" or "*union*". In the practice of yoga, we are connecting our minds and our bodies. As a traditional formal practice, there is no other goal than this union - though it can be easy to strive for something measurable like finally getting into a challenging posture. In both yoga and body scan, we are interfacing our awareness and attention through *sense-felt* experiences of the body that are arising here and now.

Along with the breath, we are now including the sensations of the body. We may also discover how to consciously direct the breath (and with it our full attention) to specific regions of the body. This is the essence of Body Scan:

- Lie on the floor, or sit in a chair
- Bring awareness and attention to your breath
- Inhale and exhale first to the toes of one foot
- Progress through this foot, ankle and leg to the hip on successive breath cycles
- Repeat this sequence for the other leg
- Continue up through the rest of the body

Jon Kabat-Zinn has produced a guided body scan meditation that is available as CD or downloadable format through his Mindfulness-Based Stress Reduction program.

There are numerous forms of yoga offered world-wide. Choose a gentle and simple form that will support you in the practice of mindfulness. The intent is to train consistent awareness-attention-interface through the "here-

and-nowness" of breathing and sense-felt experience. Again, we are blessed with bodies that exist only here and now.

Over forty years ago, I began to explore yoga and self-guided body scan. At that time, my attention-mind was like a wild banshee, as my awareness slumbered. I lived with constant stress and acute anxiety caused by my rampant and unchecked mind. At 18 years of age, I was aging fast - suffering from chronic stress and my inability to embrace that stress and use it as a vector for fitness.

In the ensuing four-plus decades, I have slowly crafted these simple practices into highly effective deep processes that are integral to my life. I continue to practice a form of body scan almost daily: After my morning training, I often lay down and circulate my breath through my body. This mindfulness practice has become a highly effective form of "active" recovery. I also use this *during* multi-day ultra triathlons - pausing for 10-20 minutes to lay down and recharge.

I practice a blend of yoga and Pilates at least twice a week that serves both as mindfulness practice and functional strength training. In my experience these two are interrelated - again, something I refer to as *intelligent* functional strength. I attribute my long-term freedom from injury to both the mindfulness skills and the functional strength I derive from this formal practice.

Simple T'ai Chi: I practice a slow-moving meditative form of T'ai Chi every morning when I arise. (The Chinese call it *playing* T'ai Chi.) To really emphasize proprioception and my sense-felt experience, I practice everyday *with my eyes closed*. I also focus on synchronizing the inhale and exhale of each breath with specific movements. In my experience this is an essential part of the practice to activate and circulate chi energy.

While I have been practicing this same sequence of moves for most of my life now, most times I practice - with a curious Beginner's Mind - I discover and experience something deeper and more profound than any previous time. The circulation and orchestration of chi energy continues to get stronger and more articulate. (By the way, my unfailing, faithful and reliable guide throughout this decades-long exploration is gravity.)

"Supreme Ultimate" - this is one of the translations for *"T'ai Chi"*. I am unable to express just how deep and how powerful the daily practice of T'ai Chi has been for me over the past forty years - as an endurance athlete yes, but even more so as a healthy, balanced human being. This daily practice is simply the strongest investment I have made in my life.

While I regard T'ai Chi as the most effective way to develop proprioceptive acuity and to train mindfulness, it can take years to learn the long, elaborate sequence of movements and to make them PAGES. Years ago, when I was teaching T'ai Chi, I gave up on trying to teach a traditional long sequence of movements and chose to teach selected short segments of movements from the form, repeating them over and over. Eventually, I produced a video that enables athletes to learn these simple movements quickly. The audio narrative also provides guidance on how to breathe with each movement - an essential element often overlooked by many teachers. (The video is available through the Total Immersion website at this link.)

To summarize, in my experience of playing T'ai Chi as a mindfulness practice, it matters not whether the movements are accurate to some ancient traditional form. Far more important is the synchronicity of breath with movement, the alliance with gravity, and the interface of awareness and attention. Just ten minutes a day can improve mindfulness and health. (My practice is about 45 minutes each day.)

Approach As a Formal Practice

As goal-oriented athletes, it can be a daunting challenge for us to really *pause* and sharpen our axe of perceptive acuity through a traditional formal practice of mindfulness like sitting meditation, or T'ai Chi. Our drive is to go after the prize: We would rather attack the tree with a dull axe, a sledge hammer, or anything else that is available, rather than pause long enough to sharpen the axe.

This is why we explored Approach earlier as a prerequisite to each training session. This is why I encourage you to log the five or ten minutes of Approach time as part of your training session: It *is* part of your training session!! As master athletes, interfacing our awareness and attention is an essential part of our kaizen-durance training. That 5-10 minutes of Approach will yield much greater dividends than 5-10 additional minutes of mindless training.

If you are consistent in pausing before each training session - *even for a few minutes* - to orchestrate some way of sharpening your axe, you will begin to "own" the process - crafting your unique form of Approach. Regardless of each individual's process, the common element we all share in our Approach is to *pause* - that is, to stop doing and to simply Be Here Now. Remember:

- Beginner's Mind: no past.

- Finalist's Mind: no future.

- We only live in this present moment.

While the Approach to an endurance training session is not a traditional formal mindfulness practice, if we truly pause and "*stop doing*", it can serve us well as a formal practice:

- We are deliberate and clear in our intent to prime our perceptive acuity.

- We are not striving to accomplish anything else other than to pause and interface our awareness and attention to Be Here Now.

- We engage both Beginner's and Finalist's Mind.

- We generously invest our awareness and attention in this moment as our golden opportunity, just as it is arising.

- We summon our patience, curiosity, even our creativity.

- We bring our focus to the craft of kinetic intelligence - whether we are preparing for high-intensity intervals or an easy recovery session.

- We approach our training session with conscious breath, a relaxed, alert body, an inquisitive and patient mind, and proprioceptive awareness.

While our method of Approach to each training session is not an ancient traditional practice, it is formal: We are pausing to Be Here Now and to sharpen the axe of perceptive acuity. It's worth the pause. Now we can maximize the return on our aerobic investment.

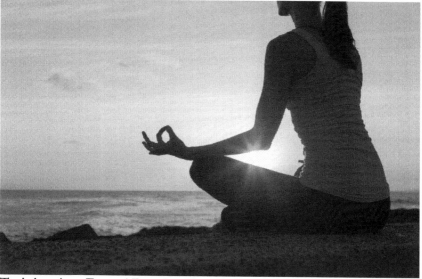

Training As a Formal Practice: Breath

In the ancient practice of sitting meditation, we exercise and engage our awareness to focus our attention on our breath. Every time our attention wanders, we exercise the awareness to return our attention to the breath. We can do *exactly the same thing* during every endurance training session - be it short or long, easy or challenging. To keep our awareness and attention on each breath, we can synchronize our breathing with our strokes/strides.

With swimming - given that our access to air is limited - we have no choice but to synchronize our breath with our strokes. It simply comes down to survival. However, we can also practice conscious breathing as we cycle, run, cross-country ski, row, etc. Sync each inhale and exhale to a specific number of strokes/strides. The number of strokes/strides per breath cycle will vary, responding to aerobic intensity and cadence.

Training As a Formal Practice: Sense-Felt Experience

PAGES movements and proprioceptive awareness demand perceptive acuity: We must craft each stroke mindfully. Our quest for effortless power advances most effectively through mindfulness training - specifically focusing on our sense-felt experience as it arises. Here are a few suggestions for sensations you can focus on as you swim, bike or run:

Swim: Really *feel* the flow of water from your fingertips to your elbow during the Entry and Extension phase of each stroke. (Imagine that you are slipping your arm into a sleeve.) You can actually close your eyes to enhance that feeling-focus. Use your attention to refine your Entry/Extension so that you disturb the water less and slip through the sleeve faster. As you improve that attention, feel the sleeve extend the from fingertips to shoulder, and then fingertips to hip, and finally all the way to your toes.

Bike: As you pedal, train your attention to your pelvic core. Feel the bowl of bone and how it pitches forward and sits on the saddle. Strive to minimize movement in the saddle - what I call "*saddle silence*". Saddle silence is essential for efficiency, stability, safety, and even *comfort* as you ride. Find the ideal pelvic pitch and low back profile that gives you the best stability *in this moment*. (It will change as you ride.) Keeping your attention here, focus on propelling your pelvic core forward - not side-to-side, or up-and-down. Maintaining attention on this subtle sense-felt experience is a real challenge with so many changing variables on the road. You can train this attention first on a stationary stand. Saddle silence.

Run: You can also train your attention to your pelvic core as you run. As with cycling, focus on moving your pelvic core forward - not side-to-side, or up-and-down. Unlike cycling, as you run, your core will rotate side-to-side with each stride. That rotation contributes to stride length. Like cycling, this sense-felt experience may be subtle at first.

As you run, you may instead choose to focus first on the sense-felt experience of each foot contact: The soles of our feet have lots of nerve endings that sense pressure. As you run, at the instant of initial contact, feel how and where this pressure begins in your foot. Can you anticipate exactly where and when you will first feel contact? How does that pressure spread through the sole of each foot? Where and when is the moment of greatest pressure? And where is the last moment of pressure as your foot leaves the ground? How does your foot respond to each contact: Do you tense and contract your foot, or allow it to relax and spread?

These are just a few of the *thousands* of sense-felt experiences that provide us with guidance in our quest to craft evermore PAGES movements through mindfulness. There is no limit to our experience-ability. It starts with mindfulness - a durable interface of awareness with attention fully occupying and engaging with this present moment.

Summary: Through conscious breath and sense-felt experience, our daily training sessions can constitute a significant portion of our mindfulness training. And unlike traditional formal practices that may have no obvious and immediate benefits, we are easily motivated by the mindfulness opportunities offered by endurance training to attain our goals. However, conducting endurance training sessions as a formal practice of mindfulness requires discernment: We must temper our desire and drive to attain goals and "hit those numbers" so that we will patiently craft the skills of mindfulness. Our success with this temperance is determined by our Approach.

Informal Practice

Every moment of our lives offers us an opportunity to practice mindfulness, to invest one hundred percent of our awareness and attention in this present moment as it arises. Every moment offers us an opportunity for kaizen, regardless of the circumstances. This is true across the spectrum of our day-to-day lives - from the mundane repetitive daily tasks that seem to require no skill at all, to the most momentous or dangerous events of our lives. If we find it challenging to awaken our awareness and focus our attention in the present moment during formal practice, it may feel impossible to wake up and practice mindfulness during our day-to-day - especially during low-consequence events.

What distinguishes formal from informal practice? Formal practice includes a clear intent as well as a beginning and an ending. Informal practice lacks these clear definitions.

Our daily lives are filled with obligations and responsibilities. Each day, we feel compelled to get things done just to survive. In this survival mode, it's easy to feel that there just isn't enough time or energy to approach these obligations as some kind of special opportunity for mindfulness training or kaizen. We are easily caught up in the drama and circumstance, or put off by the boredom and fatigue. When we feel violated, even in a non-threatening way - someone cuts in line ahead of us - we are swept away by our anger, our fear, our sense of entitlement.

We are not orchestrating our lives, they are happening to us. We are on the treadmill of life, and we cannot seem to control the speed. What can we do?

Pause

As master athletes, just before we train, we orchestrate our Approach to sharpen the axe of perceptive acuity. During this Approach, the most significant thing we do is to *pause* so that we can summon our awareness and attention here and now. As we gain proficiency with this *profound action of pausing*, we can sharpen the axe *almost instantly*.

Our approach does not have to be elaborate and time consuming. It doesn't even need a capital "A". With experience, we can sharpen that axe of perceptive acuity in an instant. If we can find our way to pause even briefly, it is possible to approach any moment of our lives as an opportunity worthy of our full investment. Let's consider a few of the opportunities that arise for us each day, disguised as mundane, even boring obligations:

Ho-Hum

Washing Dishes: The meal is over and everyone is satisfied. But… Behold! There is a sink full of dishes, pots and pans to wash. Step one: Pause. Breathe consciously a few times. Embrace what lies ahead. Notice any resistance or impatience you feel. Be with it as you breathe. Summon your Beginner's Mind, your Finalist's Mind. Then focus on your *craft* for washing dishes. How can you make this process flow smoothly and gracefully? Dishwashing is a great opportunity to practice mindfulness because we are working with our hands. It requires dexterity which arises from diligent sense-felt experience. Can you wash the dishes with PAGES movements? Can you be aware of each breath as you flow through the process?

Oh, you have a dishwasher? Here, your opportunity exists as the activity of rinsing the dishes and loading the dishwasher. (And you may still have the fortune of washing the pots and pans.) You can summon the same quality of mindfulness.

Housekeeping & Groundskeeping: The dog hair is building up on the carpet. The yard is turning into a meadow. Like the dishes, it's easy to regard these tasks as obstacles that stand in the way of rest and relaxation: Get 'em out of the way quickly, and with minimal investment. We all have unique ways to clean our houses and maintain the outdoor surroundings - just like we have unique methods for endurance training. Our ways of housekeeping and groundskeeping are no less worthy of craftsmanship than how we craft our swimming strokes or running strides.

Summary: Much of the "daily drudgery" of our lives - from taking out the trash to walking from the parking lot into the grocery store and down the aisles - requires that we move our bodies. Why not make *all* of our movements PAGES? Why withhold the mindfulness required for PAGES movements just for training and racing?

Transforming a mundane "pain in the ass" into a kaizen opportunity begins with that *pause,* and the subtle shift in how we approach the activity. Each time, it's our *choice:* We can go at it with the resistance, struggle and resentment of the monkey mind, or patiently seek out a dance of grace, efficiency and effortless power through the interface of awareness and attention.

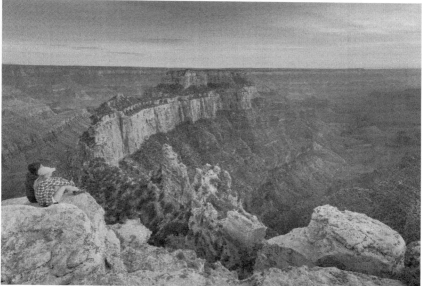

Relationships as Informal Practice

Our richest opportunities in life for kaizen - for totally interfacing and investing our awareness and attention in the present moment - arise each day in our relationships with one another. Like breathing, our relationships are a precious and vital lifeline. To say that our relationships with our loved ones or even with strangers are "informal" is misleading.

As opportunities to practice mindfulness, our relationships are "informal" because we are not accustomed to approaching and engaging with others as a mindfulness practice. We are usually preoccupied with what we want, what we feel the need to protect, or the expectations we should fulfill. We are often looking to "win", as if we are in the fighting ring. Mostly, we forget to pause.

Let's return to the wise old martial arts master. He "embraces" each opponent with his full awareness and attention, disengaging from any agendas to dominate or control. His intention is to perceive all that arises, and to seek ways to create harmony through what is arising. He embraces the Paradox of Control.

Healthy, functional relationships arise through clear and accurate perception and expression. When we approach our relationships distracted by personal agendas - desires, fears, judgments, assumptions and prejudices - we cloud and distort our perceptions. Can we really perceive what is true for others, what they are experiencing? How well do we actually *listen?*

We interact with other human beings constantly, every day. We have the opportunity each time to pause and invest our awareness and attention by really and truly *listening* to what others are communicating - through gestures as well as words. Listening is a high-level practice of mindfulness. It requires great discernment and skill to distinguish our own thoughts and feelings from what someone else is expressing. So often we misinterpret communication because we distort it with our own "stuff" - our own point of view.

It is well beyond the scope of this introductory book to explore our interrelationships as a rich domain for kaizen. Above all other forms of mindfulness practice, relationships require specific *mindfulness skills*. We will identify these skills and their relevance to an array of mindfulness practices, including endurance training, racing *and relationships* in Kaizen-durance Book 3, "Training Mindfulness Skills". Until then, at least occasionally, make the choice to *listen* to what someone else is communicating and to discern her/his communication from your inner commentary about that communication. Strive to feel her/his experience through your perceptive acuity.

Don't Forget to Breathe?

To conclude this chapter, let's return to the most basic mindfulness practice: breathing. In the ancient practice of sitting meditation, we train our awareness and attention to Be Here Now simply by observing our breath: Every time we are aware that our attention has drifted from the breath, we bring it back.

Breathing is a remarkable and unique activity for us: Without breath, we die. Yet, we do not have to consciously direct the process of breathing: If we "forget" to consciously breathe, there is still a mechanism that assures we maintain that inhale-exhale cycle at an appropriate tempo to keep us alive. Whew!! That means we can sleep without dying.

Breathing can be either conscious or unconscious. Balance is similar: We can maintain our alliance with gravity without much conscious direction. However, directing our consciousness to breath and balance can enhance the quality of each. We have already considered this with our PAGES movements: Training and improving conscious proprioception as part of our *craft* is a fundamental element of PAGES strokes and strides.

We also have the opportunity to *craft our breath*. We have that opportunity each moment of our lives. Through the craft of breathing, we can:

- Improve our health and energy

- Use conscious breath to stay present with our experience as it is - instead of resisting and reacting.

When we are present with our experience as it is, we can *respond.* - just as the Sensei responds to his opponent with grace and ease rather than reacting with fear or aggression. Response enables us to progress through the Fitness Cycle (Stress-Recovery-Adaptation) so that we grow and increase fitness. Reaction keeps us caught in the Stress phase, without orchestrating Recovery and Adaptation. This leads to dis-ease.

Conscious breath becomes our capacity to *pause* in an instant - with no elaborate process or specific circumstances - so that we can choose to approach what is occurring here and now with all of our awareness and attention.

Mindfulness begins with the most basic activities of our lives - pausing, breathing and moving.

Chapter Summary

We can pursue lifelong improvement in any area of life by training perceptive acuity. Mastery arises as we accurately perceive what is unfolding here and now. Perceptive acuity enables us to respond brilliantly. We improve perceptive acuity through mindfulness training.

At the most stripped-down, bare-bones level, we can express mindfulness practice in three one syllable words: BE HERE NOW. To sharpen the axe of perceptive acuity, we must train our awareness and attention to be here in this present moment - regardless of what is occurring. This is called *mindfulness training.*

Sitting meditation is the most effective ancient practice of training mindfulness. The training in this practice is simple: Sit quietly and focus on your breathing. When you are aware that your attention has drifted to something else, gently return to your breathing. In meditation, we are not really training that wandering "monkey mind". We are awakening and training a calm, still and subtle awareness that is "outside" our monkey mind - an awareness that can gently bring that monkey mind back to the simple here and now of our breathing.

It is natural for us to feel a strong aversion to sitting meditation. We don't seem to accomplish anything when we just sit and observe the breath. Our monkey mind can feel threatened and caged.

We have an opportunity to hone mindfulness skills every moment of our lives - either through formal or informal practice. In formal practice, simply *being here now* is our primary intention and objective - with no other motive or purpose. Traditional formal practice *is the most effective way* to acquire mindfulness skills so that we can interface our awareness and attention and sharpen perceptive acuity.

On the other hand, with informal practice, we can approach any activity as an opportunity to invest our full awareness and attention in what is arising. There is no formal context, no deliberate or explicit mindfulness preparation as we engage in the activities of the day. Through informal practice, we are embracing each moment, as it arises - ordinary or extraordinary - as the *only opportunity we have right now* to engage with and to train mindfulness.

Truly, this is the only moment we have to live in - we cannot live in the past or in the future.

Sitting meditation, yoga, body scan, and T'ai Chi are all practical forms of traditional mindfulness training. With yoga, body scan and T'ai Chi, we use the "here-and-nowness" of our body's sense-felt experience, as well as the breath, to train our awareness and attention. Each of these also offers restorative benefits for our bodies - aiding in recovery and balanced health.

As master athletes, a deliberately orchestrated Approach to each training session can also serve as a formal way of training mindfulness. In the pause of our Approach, we:

- Interface our awareness with our attention.

- Set a deliberate and clear intent to prime our perceptive acuity.

- Are not striving to accomplish anything else other than to pause and Be Here Now.

- Engage both Beginner's and Finalist's Mind.

- Generously invest in this moment as our golden opportunity, just as it is arising.

- Summon our patience, curiosity, even our creativity.

- Bring our focus to the craft of kinetic intelligence - whether we are preparing for high-intensity intervals or an easy recovery session.

- Approach the training session with conscious breath, a relaxed, alert body, an inquisitive and patient mind, and proprioceptive awareness.

As with the traditional forms of mindfulness training, we can awaken our awareness and train our attention with breath and sense-felt experience. We can train with conscious breath by synchronizing each breath cycle to a specific number of strokes or strides. There are thousands of sense-felt experiences we can draw upon for mindfulness training during each training session. We craft PAGES movements by responding to our sense-felt experience as it arises. Proprioception is a complex part of our sense-felt experience.

Conducting endurance training sessions as a formal practice of mindfulness requires discernment: We must temper our desire and drive to attain goals and "hit those numbers" so that we can patiently craft the skills of mindfulness through PAGES.

Every moment of our lives offers us an opportunity for kaizen, to invest one hundred percent of our awareness and attention in this present moment as it arises, regardless of the circumstances. However, it can be a real challenge to "wake up" and practice mindfulness during our day-to-day - especially during low-consequence events, or when we feel rushed. It's easy to feel that there just isn't enough time or energy to approach the obligations or our daily lives as opportunities to train mindfulness.

If we can find our way to *pause* even briefly before each of those pressing obligations or mundane tasks, it is possible to approach any moment and circumstance of our lives as an opportunity worthy of our full investment. We can start with mundane daily obligations like washing dishes, cleaning, groundskeeping, laundry. All of these tasks require that we move our bodies. Why not make *all* of our movements PAGES? Why withhold the mindfulness required for PAGES movements just for training and racing? Let's maximize the return on our investment in every area of our lives.

Transforming a mundane "pain in the ass" into a kaizen opportunity begins with that *pause,* and the subtle shift in how we approach each activity through the interface of awareness and attention. Each time, it's our *choice*: We can go at it with the resistance, struggle and resentment of untamed monkey mind and a sense of entitlement, or patiently seek out a dance of grace, efficiency and effortless power through the interface of awareness and attention.

Our richest opportunities in life for kaizen arise each day in our relationships with one another. Like breathing, our relationships are a precious and vital lifeline. As opportunities to practice mindfulness, our relationships are "informal" because we are not accustomed to approaching and engaging with others as a mindfulness practice. We are usually preoccupied with achieving a specific result or outcome each time we interact with someone. However, this attachment can distort our perceptions of one another.

Healthy, functional relationships arise from clear and accurate perception and expression. We have the opportunity each time we interact with someone - with *anyone* - to "pause" and clearly choose to invest our full awareness and attention by really *listening* to what others are communicating - through gestures as well as words. Listening is a high-level practice of mindfulness. It requires great discernment and skill to distinguish our own thoughts and feelings from what someone else is expressing.

We can progress along the kaizen path in our relationships by training our listening skills each time we interact with someone - from our closest companions to complete strangers.

Breathing is a remarkable and unique activity for us: Breathing can be either conscious or unconscious. Balance is similar: We can maintain our alliance with gravity without much conscious direction. However, directing our consciousness to breath and balance can enhance the quality of each.

Each moment, we have the opportunity to craft our breath and our movements - not just during formal practice and endurance training.

Conscious breath empowers us to *pause* in an instant - with no elaborate process or specific circumstances - so that we can choose to approach what is occurring here and now with all of our awareness and attention. This ability to pause and this capacity to interface our awareness and attention to what is occurring here and now are the ground from which our *brilliance* arises.

In Kaizen-durance Book 5 "Brilliance and Flow State", we will look deeply at how to reliably and consistently orchestrate brilliance and flow state in our day-to-day lives.

What's Next?

In the final chapter we summarize this introduction to kaizen-durance. We look closer at the true essence of kaizen-durance: How does our formal training as master athletes empower us in *all* areas of our lives?

CHAPTER EIGHT:

THE POWER OF CHOICE

The Power Of Choice

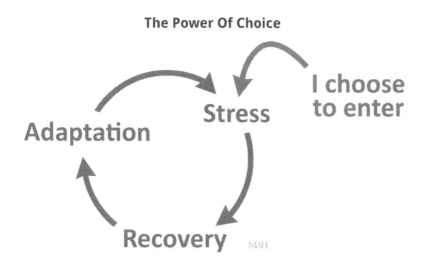

The Power of Choice

In this introductory book, we have explored the foundational elements of Kaizen-durance and how we can forge skills for lifelong improvement from these foundations. In every area of life - from sport to family to occupation - it all begins with our *choice*. As athletes, we first begin to recognize and exercise this choice when we patiently pursue mastery through kinetic intelligence, rather than relentlessly banging our heads against the aerobic wall.

As we make that choice, we become master athletes. Sure, we can still pursue goals and great performances. However, we wisely balance those sporting goals with a diligent pursuit of our endurance *craft*. Specifically, we turn our focus to crafting PAGES movements in every training session - from the easiest recovery session to the most challenging interval session.

This is a choice we exercise in each moment - not just once. And we exercise this choice with the joy of knowing there are no limits - no limits in our power to choose, no limits to the rewards we can enjoy by exercising our power of choice.

We are exercising our choice to:

- De-emphasize the diminishing resource of our aerobic capacity

- Embrace the abundant resource of our kinetic intelligence

- Transform our experience of competition from "You against me" to "A successful petition for the empowerment of companionship"

We choose to stop resisting and instead to "go with the flow". That is, we embrace the Paradox of Control:

- We give up trying to change what is arising that is beyond our control

- We tap into the flow of the forces that are arising in the moment

- We orchestrate those forces

Picture a big wave surfer. It is absurd and dangerous for the surfer to resist or attempt to change the massive wall of water that will very soon tumble and crash. Instead, the surfer rides the wave *exactly as it is* and uses the immense power to execute graceful moves - moves that are PAGES. As master athletes, we strive to ride the big wave of gravity all the way to the finish line. And we can strive to adapt our surfing skills to every area of our lives.

In this final chapter, we explore the relevance and the power of choice and how it orients our destiny - in life as well as sport. Exercising choice moment-to-moment is how we embrace the Paradox of Control:

- We cannot choose or control the circumstances that arise in our lives.

- We do however - in each moment - choose to either react or respond as those circumstances arise in our lives.

- When we choose to respond by embracing the opportunity for kaizen that exists in this moment, we can tap into the forces that are arising.

- As we tap into those forces we can experience the effortless power of going with the flow.

- Our choice to react and resist or to respond and embrace determines our destiny - beginning with our health.

Fitness Cycle

In this introductory book, we began our exploration with the Fitness Cycle: Stress-Recovery-Adaptation. We recognize now that this Fitness Cycle applies to our growth-fitness in all areas of life, not just aerobic fitness. Our success at orchestrating this cycle in any area of life is largely determined by our choice:

- Can we embrace the stressful experiences of our lives as opportunities for growth?

- Are we willing to invest our full awareness and attention in this moment as it is arising - even if we do not "like" the circumstances?

- Can we relinquish our attachment to our goals in life (like the finish line result of a race) and instead patiently focus on the process (the journey)?

Again, this Fitness Cycle is at play in *every area of our lives* - not just athletics. Cycling through the Stress-Recovery-Adaptation sequence can lead to *life* fitness, as well as athletic fitness. Our success at navigating this sequence in each moment is truly determined by our choice.

Each time we lace up our shoes and head out the door for a training session, we are ready to accept the stress of the run as an opportunity to cultivate endurance fitness. We do this by:

- Clearly choosing to orchestrate that stress by running mindfully

- Responding wisely by orchestrating adequate and appropriate recovery and adaptation.

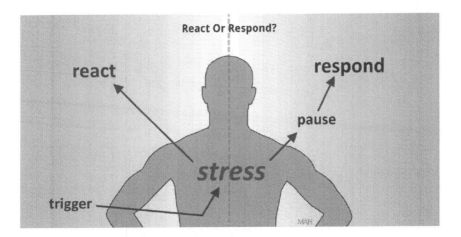

The Big Question is…

In our daily lives, as we experience stress, *do we exercise the same clear choice* to "roll the wheel" of the Fitness Cycle forward for growth and empowerment as we do with our athletic training?

Do we choose to *react* to the stresses we experience, or do we choose to *respond*? What's the difference?

> **Reaction** often arises as resistance, as *"You're doing this to me!"* or *"No, this isn't what I want! Why me?"*. Resistance prevents us from progressing through the Fitness Cycle. We get stuck at Stress, and it becomes chronic.

> **Response** arises when we recognize and accept the opportunity for growth as we are experiencing stress, and choose to invest of our awareness and attention. This investment empowers us to respond brilliantly, enabling us to move from Stress to Recovery to Adaptation.

There is a stark difference in the results you get from each attitude:

- Do you try to avoid stress? (Good luck with that!) To the extent that you are successful, there is no potential for growth.

- Do you resist and push back at the stressors in your life? This requires additional energy, creating additional stress and disrupts the fitness cycle. It prevents you from moving to the Recovery Phase. Without a balance between stress and recovery, there will be no adaptation for growth.

Pursuing Mastery: Moment-by-Moment

We experience and enjoy lifelong improvement as we patiently pursue mastery. To pursue mastery, we sharpen the axe of perceptive acuity. Each moment of our lives offers us an opportunity to sharpen that axe. It's up to us. It's our choice. We develop perceptive acuity as we choose to:

- Generously invest our awareness and attention in this moment.

- Disengage from our judgments, attachments, fears, desires, etc. - even though they may arise.

- Embrace the Paradox of Control: Give up our attachment to a result and simply focus on what is occurring here and now.

- Recognize the opportunities that are arising here and now, and the forces that are "at play".

Our capacity to perceive and to express - that is, our experience-ability - is infinite. How much of this infinite resource are we willing to invest right now? And for how long? There are no limits, and no expiration dates. This is how we pursue mastery, moment-by-moment. It's up to us. It's our choice.

The most powerful choice we can make in our lives arises in each moment: "*Am I willing to Be Here Now?*"

Approach

Approach is difficult to define, because it's not really tangible or measurable. And, it's both a noun and a verb. As a process and as an action, it is the "real thing" - the bare bones process of *pausing to choose*. In that pause, we choose to interface and invest our full awareness and attention in this present moment as it is arising. We arrive here and now with a sharp axe. (Well, why not? It's the only opportunity we have *right now* anyway.)

We have explored some techniques that can facilitate us to approach each endurance training session with a seamless interface of awareness and attention so that we can maximize the return on our aerobic investment. We can use similar techniques in any moment of our lives, so that we maximize return on our "*life investment*".

It doesn't really require any special ritual or elaborate process to pause and make a clear and deliberate choice - though these actions may be effective.

In just an instant, we can pause and choose to:

- Turn off the "auto-pilot".

- Interface our awareness and attention.

- Summon up our infinite experience-ability.

However, when we first begin to purposefully orchestrate our approach, it may require some time to pause and considerable energy to summon that awareness and attention. As an illustration, when a novice registers for that first marathon, it requires considerable training and preparation. On the other hand, a veteran who runs multiple marathons annually will require less training and preparation. The difference between the novice and the veteran? The veteran has acquired more *navigational skills* to pursue the goal through a graceful, efficient and masterful process - through mindfulness.

The words "*approach*" and "*pursuit*" both imply moving forward towards some specific destination. With tools and skills for navigation, we are more able to find and move along the path that leads us to better health, more harmony and happiness. That path may not be the most direct to reach the external goal (like a faster time). Rather, we navigate a healthy path towards deeper internal goals first (like PAGES movements that may yield that faster time) - what I call the "*path of least resistance*".

These navigational skills and our ensuing approach are subtle, intangible, and difficult to measure. The navigational skills that serve us best in our kaizen lives are the skills of mindfulness. These require diligence, commitment and perseverance to master. The process of kaizen begins over and over again in each arising moment through the rigor of choice. Can we hold that choice in our awareness moment-to-moment?

Mind IN Matter

As master athletes, we approach our goal and our practice with a sharp perceptive axe. However, our priority is no longer to attain that goal at any cost: We don't swing the axe wildly at everything in front of us as we forge on. Instead, each swing of the axe is deliberate and purposeful. We choose to pursue the goal through precision, alignment, grace, efficiency and seamless continuity. We choose the finesse of well-crafted strides and strokes, rather than the brute force of desperate exertion. We swing the axe skillfully.

Ours is a masterful choice of mind *in* matter, rather than the foolish choice of mind over matter. Honoring the sense-felt intelligence of our bodies through mind *in* matter, it probably won't require ten thousand repetitions to master a movement skill. If we are patient in the beginning, if we are willing to *start where we are* - rather than where we want to be or think we should be - we can master a skill much faster.

Patience to Pause

Here's another paradox: If we are patient enough to pause in the beginning, we can improve and progress towards our goals faster. It all starts with our choice to pause and sharpen the axe, and then to approach the goal patiently, with precision, alignment, grace, efficiency and a seamless interface of awareness and attention, of body and mind.

PAGES enable us to train and race as master athletes. Beyond our sport, we can embody these same qualities in our occupations, our relationships, our creative endeavors, even our mundane domestic chores. The choice is ours - in each moment.

Again, the question is: Can we pause and choose to summon and invest our full awareness and attention to what is arising in this moment? Each moment of our lives is a golden opportunity to practice PAGES in both our actions and our speech.

Effortless Power

Effortless power is another paradox: How can power be effortless? We can experience effortless power when we perceive and tap into the forces that are at play in the present moment. However, these forces are often difficult to detect. Gravity is a great example: We cannot see it, hear it, taste it, smell it or touch it. Yet we can always feel it within our bodies and observe it's effect on things around us... if we train our awareness and attention.

Effortless power is not the same as laziness: It turns out that effortless power is not effortless after all. Perceiving and orchestrating subtle (yet powerful) forces requires tremendous awareness and attention - and not just for a moment: We must vigilantly sustain our investment of awareness and attention. If we tap into a powerful force and then drift into auto-pilot, we will lose touch with that force. And there may be negative repercussions when our actions are unattended.

We can gain physical ease by sharpening the axe of perceptive acuity. That requires diligence, patience and investment. As master athletes, our capacity for these is far greater than our capacity for physical exertion.

Proprioceptive training as part of our kaizen-durance craft can yield direct and tangible benefits in our athletic performances as we tap into the power of gravity. Proprioceptive training is also highly effective as mindfulness training - rigorously exercising our choice to invest awareness and attention moment-to-moment, over and over again.

And finally…

Mindfulness

The ancient traditional mindfulness practice of sitting meditation is simple, stark, even austere. There is no activity more basic than:

- Sitting still and observing our breath.

- Bringing our attention back to the breath every time we are aware that it has wandered.

Sitting meditation is perhaps the most rigorous exercise of *choice:*

The choice to pause, to suspend activity and be still.

The choice to summon full awareness and attention to this moment - be it unremarkable and ordinary, or challenging, threatening or rewarding.

The choice to be present with whatever discomforts arise - physically, mentally, emotionally.

The choice to return the monkey mind to the "here and now" every time it wanders.

As I mentioned earlier, I have practiced T'ai Chi as my traditional form of mindfulness practice for the past 4 decades. While it is not as simple and direct as sitting, it serves well as a rigorous exercise in choice. I encourage you to explore traditional mindfulness practices and adapt something that feels right for you. Traditional forms of mindfulness training strengthen our awareness of the continuous moment-to-moment choice that arises over and over again.

Unlike our endurance training, traditional forms of mindfulness training are free of the distractions and desires of a finish line, a medal, or grandeur. In our daily lives, as the choice arises moment-to-moment, we must exercise that choice without the prospect of glorious recognition we often enjoy as athletes. Traditional forms of mindfulness training prepare us best to exercise our power of our choice in every moment - even those that are mundane and ordinary.

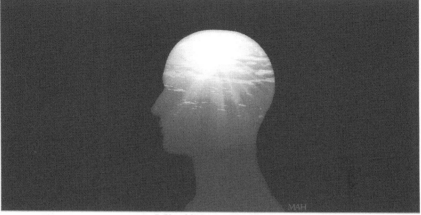

Mindfulness Skills

We can best prepare for any endeavor in our lives by acquiring a set of skills that will empower us to embrace and respond to the challenges we encounter along the way. The skills that best serve us as master athletes are *mindfulness skills*.

We have explored the benefits of PAGES as skills that can compensate for the decline of aerobic capacity as we age. Kinetic intelligence serves as a form of wisdom for us. PAGES skills arise from mindfulness skills. Jon Kabat-Zinn, Founder of the widely acclaimed Mindfulness-Based Stress Reduction, has identified and described nine *"attitudes of mindfulness"*:

- Beginner's Mind

- Trust

- Patience

- Non-Judging

- Letting Go

- Non-Striving

- Acceptance

- Gratitude

- Generosity

None of these attitudes appear particularly "athletic" or glamorous on the surface. They certainly don't appeal to our gladiator view of sport. However, these are the skills that empower us best to exercise our choice in each moment of our lives. These are the skills that help us to *navigate* the path of kaizen. We explore these in depth in Kaizen-durance Book 3 "Training Mindfulness Skills".

Action: Journal

What makes choice such a difficult course of "action"? It's so damn subtle!! It's so easy to get lost in the drama of our lives, to focus on our goals, to be driven by our fears or swept away by our judgments. When we are immersed in these real and tangible things, the subtle but profound power of choice can be undetectable to us. We simply forget to pause and sharpen the axe. We forget over and over again, day after day, year after year.

How can we wake up and be aware moment-to-moment of our choice? We need to bring *tangibility* to the actions of:

- Pausing to interface our awareness with our attention

- Investing them in what is arising here and now.

We can bring that tangibility to this subtle process by keeping a journal.

You may already be keeping a daily log or journal to record your training sessions - something we explored early on. Typically, we focus on logging our training sessions in that journal - the length of the run, what swim drills and intervals we did in the pool, the average power output on the bike. We are recording the specifics about the *stress* phase of the Fitness Cycle.

I also suggested that you begin to track what you are doing proactively for recovery and how well you recover - so that you are more aware of the balance and the progression of your Fitness Cycle. Through this journal, you are gaining awareness and skills to orchestrate that Fitness Cycle so that you can maximize return on your aerobic investment.

Are you ready to tap into your greatest power - the power of your *choice?* You can begin by journaling about the other forms of stress you experience in your life and how you are *choosing* to orchestrate the Fitness Cycle outside of sport:

- The Fitness Cycle always begins with stress as the essential vector for growth.

- Briefly describe a specific experience of stress from your daily life, what occurred and whether you chose to react or to respond to that stress. These stressors may arise through your relationships and family life, your job, your hectic schedule, your health.

- Journal about many different forms of stress: Remember, like it or not, all forms of stress are vectors for growth... or "dis-ease".

- This exercise in reflecting will encourage you to pause and (at least in hindsight) to look at the choices you make to either react or respond when the stresses arise and to distinguish between reaction and response.

- It will aide you to evaluate your approach: That is, did you exercise your choice to pause and interface your awareness and attention so that you could tap the growth potential of that stress, or did you react and push back?

- What were the thoughts, emotions and/or sensations that you experienced during the experience? Did you resist them, or did you "dive in" and really explore them?

- If you deliberately chose to embrace the experience as an opportunity for growth and fitness, what were the tools you used to navigate that choice?

- Regardless of whether you "liked" the outcome or not, can you identify any way in which you benefitted by successfully orchestrating the Fitness Cycle?

You can use this training journal as a way to identify the opportunities for training your power of choice and to guide and document how you train your "choice fitness" process in the same way you use your training journal to guide and document how you train your endurance fitness process. It may empower you to approach more of the experiences and events of your life as opportunities for fitness and the pursuit of mastery.

Journaling: At-a-Glance Recap

In your journal, write about how you:

- Pause

- Recognize and honor the opportunity that arises

- Exercise your power of choice: Respond or react?

- Invest your awareness and attention

- Tap into the forces that are arising and "surf the wave"

• Move from stress to recovery to adaptation

Summary

Choice... This is the hard-core essence, the heart and soul of kaizen. This is how we *source* and *navigate* the path of lifelong improvement reliably and consistently, through the good times and the bad. There's no glamour, no fanfare, no immediate gratification or recognition. Choice is the deepest form of exercise and training.

Our daily zendurance training sessions - along with any form of traditional formal mindfulness practice - provide us with clear opportunities to repeatedly exercise our choice to Be Here Now. As we gain familiarity with the landscape of choosing to Be Here Now, we gain the skills to exercise our choice in any and every moment of our lives. While this approach can improve our athletic performances, the greatest benefit to us and to those around us arises in our everyday lives - our relationships, occupations, etc.

It's up to us. It's our choice.

What's Next?

In this introductory book, we have briefly explored a paradigm shift of the "how" and "why" of endurance sports for aging athletes. I have offered some basic tools to assist you in using your passion and discipline for endurance training to navigate a kaizen path for mastery and lifelong improvement - in sports and in every area of life.

If this paradigm and this kaizen approach resonates with you, I welcome and encourage you to *read on!* I am writing four more books that offer deeper insight and guidance to further your craft as an athlete and your mastery in life. These four books are sequential - building one to the next.

Book 2: *"A Guide to Neural Fitness: The Foundation for KI"*

For decades, exercise physiology has honed the science of metabolic training (also known as aerobic system training) to precision methods and mathematical formulas that can be implemented for peak performance.

Book Two boldly explores a potential of exercise physiology that has seen very little scientific attention at all – the fledgling science of *neural fitness*. I have devoted the past four decades to the study of neural fitness and its application to endurance sports. Training neural fitness is the secret to a successful "Kinetic Intelligence Hack".

Book 3: "Training Mindfulness Skills"

This may seem like a very dry and sedate subject for endurance athletes. However, mindfulness skills are the essential navigational tools for kaizen-durance: for training neural fitness, acquiring kinetic intelligence and truly maximizing your return. The good news is that you can train these skills while you are training for endurance. Your zendurance approach - that is, your mindful approach to training and racing - will enhance your athletic performance and your "life fitness".

In this book we consider each of the nine "attitudes" that Jon Kabat-Zinn has identified. We explore the opportunities in our zendurance training to develop each of them, as well as the opportunities that arise in our daily lives. Developing these mindfulness skills is the most effective way to maximize the return on our aerobic investment.

Book 4: "A Guide to Neural Training: Building KI in Your Daily Workouts"

We delve into the specifics of structuring and executing neurally-based training for endurance athletes – at any age, at any fitness or experience level. Neurally-based training sessions are the day-by-day process of hacking your athletic performance potential. We don't need to ignore or compromise conventional metabolic training to embrace and implement neural training. These two processes can be compatible, even as our focus changes to prioritize neural training over metabolic. For both approaches, the training objectives are still endurance, strength and speed. We can design and structure sessions that will improve both metabolic and neural fitness *simultaneously*. However, when we target neural training as the priority, we also accelerate kinetic intelligence.

This book provides guidelines for designing and structuring neural training sessions to focus on endurance, strength, speed, recovery *and kinetic intelligence*. Includes drills and exercises to improve neuromuscular function and performance for swim, bike and run. It is important to note that Books 2 and 3 are vital prerequisites to Book 4.

Book 5: "A Guide to Triangulating Awareness: Your GPS for Life"

In our hi-tech world, GPS units are everywhere - in our phones, on our wrists, in our cars, on our bikes. All of these operate by *triangulation:* A GPS unit receives signals from *three* satellites and then compares them to determine location, orientation (direction of travel) and velocity. GPS won't work if we can only reference one or two satellites.

There is another "GPS system" that each of us has free and unlimited access to. It is a universal and one-hundred-percent-reliable GPS system that we can use at any time to navigate the "landscape" of our lives. Each of us has unlimited access to *three aspects of consciousness*. In Book 5, we examine these three aspects and, as individuals, evaluate the strength of our personal connection to each. We explore ways to improve our balance and triangulation with these three aspects of consciousness to create the most powerful "GPS" of all. We discover how to use this personal "life-fitness GPS system" to navigate the kaizen path in any experience that arises in our lives.

Book 6: "Brilliance and Flow State"

Mastery arises as *brilliance* - something that can't be contrived, or bought and sold. When we enter Flow State, we experience sustained periods of brilliance. Sharing brilliance and flow state with others is empowering, exhilarating and healing. In Book 6, we look at the nature of brilliance and how the pursuit of mastery arises as brilliance. We go on to discover how we can orchestrate the phases of flow state so that we can consistently and reliably enjoy *and share* sustained brilliance in any and every life experience.

ABOUT THE AUTHOR

Shane Eversfield is Founder and C.E.W.* of Kaizen-durance. A degree in Modern Dance, 40 years of T'ai Chi practice and a lifelong passion for mindful movement and "kinetic intelligence" fuel his innovative fusion study of applied kinesiology and mindfulness. As an athlete, author, educator, artist and coach, he has earned the respect of many endurance athletes and coaches the world over.

Eversfield teaches over 200 classes and clinics every year in swimming, cycling, running and Kaizen Skills. He has trained and educated coaches and athletes in the US, Europe and Asia. He is based out of Island Health and Fitness in Ithaca, NY, and is a staff coach for the Total Immersion Swim Studio in New Paltz, NY.

Now 60+ years young, he continues his personal Kaizen path and the cultivation of kinetic intelligence through his daily endurance arts practice. He enjoys multi-day triathlons and ultra running events each year. and continues to quietly slip past his perceived limits. Shane regards himself as a modern-day "traditional" martial artist – deeply committed to the craft of mindful movement – rather than an as athlete.

Visit https://kaizen-durance.com/ for information about:

– Kaizen-durance® Endurance Arts Camps, Clinics, Classes: Locally (Ithaca, NY) and internationally
– Kaizen Skills: Fitness for Your Life Programs
– Bio for Shane Eversfield, Founder and C.E.W.* of Kaizen-durance

* C.E.W.: Chief Endurance Whisperer

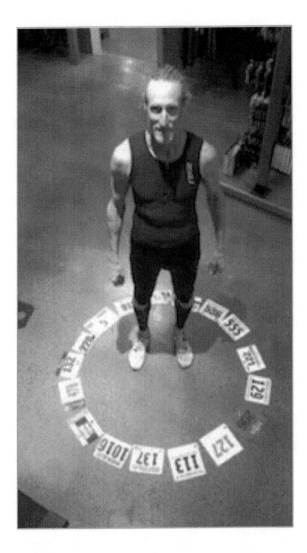

Made in the USA
Middletown, DE
30 December 2019